Baby Name Encyclopedia

The Perfect Baby Name Adviser

Sylvie Nicole

"Baby Name Encycolpedia: The Perfect Baby Name Adviser," by Sylvie Nicole. ISBN 1-58939-750-9.

Published 2005 by Virtualbookworm.com Publishing Inc., P.O. Box 9949, College Station, TX 77842, US.

Manufactured in the United States of America.

Contents

INTRODUCTION

THIS IS AN EXCEPTIONAL BOOK. It is a guide-book for all future parents helping them to choose the most appropriate name of their baby.

The book was not created easily bit I continued to write it knowing that I will help you a lot in the appropriate choice. You will enjoy yourselves, while you read it and you will select the most beautiful name for your child unnoticeably, quickly and easily, which joy will later pass onto him or her, listening to the melodious sound of his or her name.

I propose to you various categories as: Numerology for the check of the fate and the qualities of each name; analysis of the most sex appealing names; the most popular names of the new century; selection of a name according to the first letter; teams of names, meaning beauty, intellect and lots of others. The thousands of names I have selected will take you on a pleasant excursion, helping you to find out which renowned people were born on the day when your baby will be born too. The final destination is the choice of the name most intensively desired by you now. You should not forget that your child is forced to accept a name selected by other people's motives, considerations and arguments. Calling him with the appropriate name you will choose, you will help for the revival of everything he or she will represent in the future. As parents, you further to your own wish, turn out to be dependent on the tradition – family, generic, national and on the assessment, given by the bearer itself some time later on. All that exerts complex influence over the choice of the name, one or another of these factors giving superiority in the specific events. Choice is responsibility. The name must be liked not solely by you, but it should also provide the remaining close to you people with joy, and first of all it must be liked by her or by him, who will be identified by it in the society all their lives. The qualities of the name must be very carefully assessed in view of the attitude to it within the limits of seven, eight and more decades, i.e. of a whole human life. One should feel that his or her name becomes to him or her, that it is an unabolished part of him or her. The name is a combination of letters or sounds, it is the human "Self".

With this book, I want to facilitate you to make your appropriate choice and let your child grow up as an independent and unique personality. The sense of life is to give. This is why give the most beautiful name to your child. It will be his or her calling card in life.

15 Baby Name Tips

Picking a name for your new baby boy or girl is one of the most important decisions you will have to face. Remember that the name is what identifies your baby for the rest of his or her life, so choose wisely!

1. The baby name should have a positive connotation for you.

The baby name should be pleasant and meaningful. A baby name has a strong first impression. Your baby's name reflects how you picture your baby as an adult. If you imagine that he may become an athletic person, you might select a name, which reflects physical strength and athleticism.

2. The baby first name's rhythm should match the last name.

As a tip, the number of syllables in the first name should not match the number of syllables in the last name. Say the first, middle and last name several times to test the rhythm. Say the first name and last name together, too. Also, be conscious of what the first name and last name together say. If you have a common or easy to pronounce last name (i.e. Smith, Jones, Brown), you might find that an unusual or long first name can complement the last name nicely. Or as one web visitor put it, a long or unusual first name "spices up the whole name." Examples include Dakota Smith, Lucinda Brown and Sharona Flynn.

3. Check the pronunciation and spelling of the baby's name.

If you use an unusual pronunciation, your child will need to continually correct it. On the other hand, if the name is common, an unusual spelling will distinguish your child. Another factor is the ability to find personalized items. Unusual spellings will mean you have to special order or do without the personalized item.

4. The initials should not spell anything undesirable.

Check the first initial of the first and last name. Do they stand for anything? How about when you include all the middle name(s)? If the initials are not satisfactory, then the first and middle names can be switched. The child can still use the middle name on a day by day basis. For **example,** the name Paul Ivan Goldstein has the initials POG or Richard Alexander Thompson RAT.

5. Honor a family member.

Does your family have a tradition of picking names from the family tree? If this is important to you by all means stick with your family's tradition. Just remember, it is your decision so no one should have a final say on the name except you and your partner. Don't let family members coerce you into a name you do not like. You can always choose to honor a family member by using their name as a middle name.

6. Combine names to create a new baby name.

You can choose two or more words to create a unique baby name. By separating each word into syllables and combining the syllables, you can create new baby names. You can even scramble a word to create a new baby name. For **example**, Sarita can come from combining the names Sam and Rita.

7. Be conscious of nicknames and variations.

Are you prepared to hear your child called by a nickname? Andrew will inevitably become "Andy" some of the time, even if you insist on the formal name. If you like the potential nicknames associated with the name you choose, well and good. But if you have strong feelings against them, think about choosing another name with nicknames you like better or consider names without commonly used nicknames such as "Eric" or "Mary."

8. Practice the baby's name and hear how it feels.

You will say this name thousands of times. You will say lovingly and in anger. You will whisper it when the child is asleep and yell it when dinner is ready.

9. Avoid letter redundancy between names.

Often, first and last names with the same first letter do not sound well together. Also, if the last name ends with a vowel, the first name usually should not. The first name should not end with a syllable that rhymes with the first syllable of the last name. For **example**, Angela Anna has quite a few letter A's.

10. Consider the baby name´s meaning.

You may want to consider the importance of the baby name's meaning. Even if this is not important to you, it may be important to your child.

11. Is an odd baby name a good thing?

Think twice before choosing an odd baby name. Research suggests kids with odd names are teased more by peers and are overall less socialized. But if your family is full of bravado and energy, odd baby names may be a great thing.

12. Baby names are cyclical.

Baby names which were once considered old fashioned will often come back into style. 'Isaac' was a seldom used baby name for a long time, but has recently come back into fashion.

13. When to avoid celebrity baby names.

Some celebrities can become so much larger than life, their name becomes one you may not want to use for your baby name. We may never see many people naming their children Elvis or Cher.

14. Baby names using the mother's maiden name.

If retaining the mother's maiden name is important, and you do not like hyphenating last names, try using the maiden name as the first name or middle name. Many maiden names may not be best suited for a first name, but will often make a great middle name.

15. When your baby is born.

There are so many things to consider! When your baby is born, you realize it's all a matter of feeling, not logic. And your feelings and your partner's matter more than any opinion offered by friends or family. Stick with the name you genuinely love. And look forward to welcoming your child, its proud bearer.

Meanings of the First Letters

The Letter A

A = 1. A is both the first letter of the alphabet and the first vowel. It represents the head.

Determination, enterpris , courage and strength of mind: you love adventures and experiments. You aim to fulfill your fantasies. In order to be more successful, rely more on friends and relatives.

A as the first vowel in a name means the person has a strong interest in life in general, and possesses an independent nature. When another A appears in the name it brings with it the quality of being level-headed and having the ability to think problems through. When three or more A's appear in the name, this can tip the scales toward selfishness.

The negative A can be a critical and skeptical individual, looking down upon the efforts of others from their lofty place of self-righteousness.

The Letter B

B = 2. B is the second letter of the alphabet and represents the emotions. It is not a particularly strong letter on the physical plane, and can be influenced easily by others.

Super sensitiveness: you are shy, close and avoid noise parties. You have a good taste for luxury. You believe your partner is obliged to prove every day her/his feelings for you.

A love of domesticity, peace and quiet. A feminine B has a naturally motherly nature, while the male B has a love of nature and life in the country. They both feel a strong need for partnership, and have a strong dislike to being on their own. A negative B can be quite selfish, concerned with themselves and what they can get. They can also become greedy and possessive.

The Letter C

C =3 and is the third letter of the alphabet. It represents energy.

C is good-humored, extravagant and dexterous. The C is a natural talker, a born orator, with an intuitive and creative talent for eloquence. The C loves to be the organizer, and can be quite impulsive. You have infinite belief in your own abilities and you can cope with every challenge.

A negative C can be shameless, negligent, careless and unscrupulous.

The Letter D

D = 4 and is the 4th letter of the alphabet. It represents balance and organization.

Sense of duty: in most cases, you are dependable, unless you are carried away by some stupid idea and decide to follow it blindly. You are not afraid of hardships and don not comply with other people's opinions. You find it hard to express your feelings. You do not like noisy meetings and have intensified sense of the true values in life.

The negative D can be stubborn, unyielding and uncompromising in its way of looking at situations. Push it far enough, and the negative D can easily be described as pig-headed.

The Letter E

E = 5 and is both the fifth letter of the alphabet and the second vowel. It is a strong letter, representing communication.

Skilful, intellectual, imaginative and good-humored: everybody likes you for your sense of humor and optimism and admire you for taking such good care of your family.

E as the first vowel in a name points toward an interesting and event filled life. A person with 3 or more E's in their name can be nervous and temperamental, especially if E is the first vowel. A negative E can be irresponsible, unreliable and flirtatious.

The Letter F

F = 6 and is the sixth letter of the alphabet. It is a letter representing love.

Domesticated and home-loving. F is friendly, a planner, comforting and loyal. It is very easy for the F to carry a strong sense of family responsibility. The family is the most important thing for her/him.

A negative F can easily spend a lot of their time being sad, depressed and anxious; feeling a vague sense of unease, even while sitting in the midst of plenty.

The Letter G

G = 7 and is the seventh letter of the alphabet. G represents mysticism and religion.

Purposeful, orderly, inventive and instinctive. G can become quite involved with acting conventionally. Your exceptional business flair enables you to succeed in the business sphere and reach the top of the hierarchy.

The negative G loves to do things its own way. They heartily dislike advice, choosing to see it as interference. G can also be a doubter, and hard to convince of anything beyond its own, cherished opinions.

The Letter H

H = 8 and is the eighth letter of the alphabet. It represents creativity and power.

H is, by nature, successful, self-contained, and a natural money maker. It has a strong connection with the earth, and is a lover of nature. Instead of troubling you, competition motivates you even more in order to achieve your goals. Your talent of predicting the events prevents you from being surprised unpleasantly.

A negative H will be quite possessive, self-absorbed and greedy.

The Letter I

I = 9 and is the ninth letter of the alphabet, as well as being the third vowel. It represents law.

I is genteel, impulsive, elegant and has warmth of heart. I is an inspirational letter. Though you are kind, sensitive and friendly, living with you is not always easy.

I as the first vowel in a name describes a person who is interested in the arts, science and drama. A negative I can be timid, nervous and quick to become angry, or fearful. When coming from the negative aspect of their nature, I's are easily offended.

The Letter J

J = 10/1 and is the tenth letter of the alphabet. J represents aspiration.

Clever, truthful, creative and helpful. J is warm-hearted, well-meaning and reliable. You find it very hard to make your life choice.

A negative J can be lazy, listless, dull and lethargic because they have no goal in life.

The Letter K

K = 11/2, and as the eleventh letter of the alphabet, K represents extremes. This is the first of the Master Numbers.

K has a somewhat unyielding attitude to life and other people. Yet it is sensitive, vigorous and creative. K sees itself as an authority figure. You are characterized with incredible pragmatism and strong adaptability to circumstances.

The negative K can appear to be timid, fearful, nervous and miserable.

The Letter L

L = 12/3 and is the twelfth letter of the alphabet. L represents action.

L is loyal, has a natural balance, and is a good manager, along with having a kind disposition and an intellectual mind. In love, you strive not to give yourself out without receiving anything in return.

A negative L can be accident-prone, being especially vulnerable to tripping and falling.

The Letter M

M = 13/4 and is the thirteenth letter of the alphabet. M represents spirituality.

M has patience, is industrious, courageous and domesticated. The first letter of your name attracts happiness and activates your creative talent. You are capable of getting in contact with different people and make them like you.

The negative M is kind-of hasty, and behaves impatiently, or without thinking. They can also be bad tempered, and quick to anger.

The Letter N

N = 14/5 and is the fourteenth letter of the alphabet. N represents imagination.

N is very certain of itself, as a writer and spokesman. N is imaginative and loves pleasure; especially when indulging the senses. Be careful with your excessive suspiciousness human nature. They can stop your from finding a soul-mate.

A negative N can be envious, covetous and jealous, which can cause divorce or separation (in both business and personal relationships), if it is taken to extremes.

The Letter O

O = 15/6. It is both the fifteenth letter of the alphabet and the fourth vowel. O represents patience.

O brings, and carries, a sense of responsibility. It is knowledgeable and intellectual. And it can, under threatening conditions, become moral to the point of being solemn. You can complicate your life and provoke people's disapproval by behaving in an eccentric and provoking way to them.

O as the first vowel in a name reveals a frank, methodical person who has respect for law and order in everything. A negative O should guard against jealousy and learn not to wear his or her heart on the sleeve.

The Letter P

P = 16/7 and is the sixteenth letter of the alphabet. It represents power.

P is shrewd, thoughtful, talented, expressive and influential. Your sense of responsibility and discretion make you a perfect business partner.

A negative P is usually possessive, self-absorbed and with little time or sympathy for anyone else or their problems.

The Letter Q

Q = 17/8. As the seventeenth letter of the alphabet, Q represents originality.

Q has a resolute energy, is enigmatic and difficult to analyze. Q has a determined personality, it is intense, and is a natural leader. Born adventurous, you are intuitive and too self-confident.

Negative Q's are rather boring people, especially when they talk too much. They are inclined to become extremely self-centered.

The Letter R

R = 18/9 and is the eighteenth letter of the alphabet. R represents possibilities.

Enthusiastic, patient and even-tempered. R is stable, hard-working, warm hearted and compassionate.

A negative R is prone to mislaying or losing their possessions, and tends to be somewhat irritable, emotionally touchy and a bit of a miser. It is easy to aggravate a negative R, and to experience their rather short temper. Arrogance and pride can play trick on you and make you fail.

The Letter S

S = 19/1 and is the nineteenth letter of the alphabet. It represents beginnings.

S in endowed with strong feelings, and is capable of lots of effort. Attractive, and with an easy magnetism for money and finances. S brings new beginnings. S is, by nature, successful, self-contained, and a natural money maker.

A negative S may experience many upheavals and failures during their life time. They are inclined to act impulsively and without reflecting on past experiences.

The Letter T

T = 20/2 and is the twentieth letter of the alphabet. T represents growth.

T means action as well, emotion and restlessness. It is moral and religious; it has determination and is a builder. There is a natural authority to T, and it is creative. T is a very good-natured, clever and a true friend.

Negative T's are over-emotional, and easily influenced by the opinions of others. They need to learn self-control in their thoughts, words and deeds.

The Letter U

U = 21/3. U is both the twenty-first letter of the alphabet and the fifth and last "true" vowel. It represents accumulation.

U is clever and shrewd, as well as being a collector and gatherer. A fascinating character, yet hard to know. U is lucky, and it never forgets an injury, or a good deed done. You are very sensitive and you easily get disappointed.

With U as the first vowel in a name, the person it represents is capable of understanding a great deal. It also gives the ability to formulate plans and carry them out. Negative U's can be selfish, indecisive and very acquisitive.

The Letter V

V = 22/4 and is the twenty-second letter of the alphabet. It represents construction.

V is very honest and truthful, reliable and loyal. The V is gregarious, practical, industrious, sensitive and has very firm beliefs. He is also a very good friend.

A negative V can be very impractical and extremely unpredictable.

The Letter W

W = 23/5 and it is the twenty-third letter of the alphabet. It represent self-expression.

W is persistent and full of purpose. It can be hard to know, and at the same time, is charming and sociable. W is naturally attractive, affable and with imagination. People admire you because you can control yourself in crisis and when you begin some work, you finish it good.

A negative W is way too fond of taking risks and cutting corners for his/her own good. This leads to many problems for themselves and others.

The Letter X

X = 24/6. X is the twenty-fourth letter of the alphabet. It represents sexuality.

X is a born sensualist and, as such, is the natural seeker of pleasure. The X loves comfort, is easily led, and does not like to be tied down to commitment. X is an excellent money-maker and loves luxury.

A negative X can be a somewhat promiscuous person who is not only unfaithful in promises, but in their affections and commitments also.

The Letter Y

Y = 25/7 and is the 25th letter of the alphabet. Y is one of the letters in the alphabet which, under certain conditions, is also used as a vowel. It represents freedom.

Y is very much the pioneer, and can't stand being held back. It is aesthetic, independent and enterprising. Y is also generous and compassionate.

Y is classed as a vowel when it takes on the sound of either an E or an I in a name. This depends on the pronunciation, and it is given the value of the sound it emulates. For example, E as in the name Yvonne or I in the name Lynda.

A negative Y is indecisive when faced with choice. This causes them to miss much of the happiness in life.

The Letter Z

Z = 26/8 and, as the last letter in the alphabet, Z represents hope.

Z is trusting, compassionate, with a sense of consideration for other people. It is practical and down-to-earth, combined with common-sense and diplomacy. Z is very responsible person and good-hearted person.

A negative Z can be a very impatient, head-strong individual who needs to learn to think before acting or speaking.

Top 100 Most Popular Female and Male names

Rank	Male	Meaning	Rank	Female	Meaning
1	Jacob	held by the heel	1	Jessica	God's grace
2	Adam	earth, created by God	2	Emma	universal, all-embracing
3	Michael	Who is Like God	3	Ashley	Ash Tree Meadow
4	Justin	just, true	4	Brigit	resolute, strength, saint
5	Matthew	Gift of God	5	Sarah	Princess
6	Chris	Anointed, Follower of Christ	6	Christina	Anointed, Follower of Christ
7	William	valiant protector	7	Nicole	Victorious People
8	Jason	Healer	8	Jennifer	white wave, white spirit, white cheeked
9	Peter	Rock	9	Natalie	birthday, child born at Christmas
10	David	Beloved	10	Susan	Lily
11	Joshua	God Saves	11	Amy	Beloved
12	Ryan	Little King	12	Vanessa	a butterfly
13	Paul	Small, Humble	13	Amber	Yellow Gold Precious Jewel
14	Richard	Powerful, Brave Ruler	14	Victoria	victory
15	Kevin	Handsome, Gentle, Beloved	15	Michelle	Who is Like God
16	Steven	Crowned	16	Kimberly	Cyneburg's land
17	James	Supplanter, Representative	17	Amanda	Worthy of Love

18	Eric	Powerful ruler	18	Stephanie	Crowned
19	Anthony	Flower	19	Courtney	From the court
20	Thomas	Twin	20	Elisabeth	God's oath
21	Joey	God Will Increase	21	Shannon	Wise one, river name
22	Max	Greatest	22	Alison	Noble, truth
23	Brian	Noble, Strong	23	Olivia	Kind one; olive tree, peace
24	Andy	Courageous, Valiant, Man	24	Abigail	Head of a monastery, a father's joy
25	Daniel	God is My Judge	25	Kathrin	Blessed, Pure, Holy
26	Mark	warlike, hammer, defender	26	Julia	Softhaired, youthful, downy-haired, gentle
27	Christopher	Christ-bearer	27	Lindsay	Pool island, linden island
28	Brandon	fiery hill, sword	28	Marissa	Of the Sea
29	Aron	shining light, high mountain, messenger	29	Brenda	Fiery hill, sword-blade
30	Sean	God is Gracious	30	Kristen	Anointed, Follower of Christ
31	Henry	Ruler of the Home	31	Sandra	Protector of Mankind
32	Sam	God Has Heard	32	Simone	Listener
33	Nick	Victorious People	33	Kendi	Loved One
34	Dylan	sea god, son of the waves	34	Daniel	God is My Judge
35	Alexander	Protector of Mankind	35	Gabriela	Strength of God
36	Kyle	Narrow channel	36	Barbara	foreign, strange, exotic, mysterious
37	Benjamin	Son of My Right Hand	37	Carmen	garden, field of fruit, song
38	Vincent	Victorious, Conqueror	38	Melanie	Dressed in black, dark

39	Stephen	Crowned	39	Holly	Plant with red berries
40	Nicolas	Victorious People	40	Kelly	Church, warrior, wood, holly; farm by the spring
41	Charley	Manly, strong	41	Linda	Beautiful
42	Christian	Anointed, Follower of Christ	42	Hanah	Gracious
43	Nathan	Gift of God	43	Diana	Divine
44	John	God is merciful	44	Sydney	From city of St. Denis
45	Chad	Warlike, warrior	45	Valentine	Good health
46	Scott	Of Scottish Origin	46	Larissa	Name of a city, mythical woman; cheerful one
47	Craig	From near the crag	47	Stacey	Stable
48	Frank	From France, free	48	Naomi	Pleasent one; above all, beauty
49	Samuel	His name is God	49	Hillary	Cheerful
50	Dennis	Of Dionysus	50	Grace	Grace, blessing
51	Greg	Fierce	51	Angelina	Heavenly Messenger
52	Jimmy	Supplanter, Representative	52	Lauren	Laurel leaves, honour, fame, spirit
53	Dave	Beloved	53	Wendy	White, Fair
54	Bruce	Thicket, woodlands	54	Teresa	Summer, Harvester
55	Simon	Listener	55	Selena	Moon
56	Martin	Of Mars	56	Cindy	Moon, Greek god
57	Jack	God is merciful	57	Summer	Summer Season
58	Matthias	Gift of God	58	Megan	mighty, strong, able, pearl
59	Lucas	bringer of light	59	Claudia	Crippled, Lame
60	Ralph	Wise Ruler, Wolf	60	Chelsey	Landing Place
61	Andreas	Courageous,	61	Angel	Heavenly Messenger

		Valiant, Man			
62	Brad	broad meadow	62	Brandy	Brandy, Warm and Comforting Drink
63	Kale	Strong, Manly	63	Leslie	Small Meadow
64	Ben	Blessed	64	Virginia	Chaste, maiden
65	Jonathan	God Has Given	65	Margaret	Pearl
66	Roland	From famous land	66	Veronica	True image
67	Bobby	Bright Fame	67	Monica	Advice
68	Lennard	Lion hearted	68	Britney	From England, strong, industrious
69	Claude	Crippled, Lame	69	Caroline	Strong, melody, song
70	Markus	Warlike, hammer, defender	70	Sabrina	From the border land
71	Kelvin	Name of a river, from the narrow river	71	Andrea	Womanly
72	Jeremy	God will uplift, appointed by God	72	Rachel	Little Lamb, an ewe, one with purity
73	Lee	Cow, weary one, glad tidings, mistress, ruler	73	Daisy	Day's eye, flower name
74	Kenneth	Handsome, Fiery	74	Kylie	Boomerang
75	Rick	Powerful, Brave Ruler	75	Ariel	Lioness of God
76	Oliver	Olive Tree	76	Mackenzie	Son of the wise leader
77	Manuel	God is With Us	77	Marta	Warlike
78	Bernhard	Bold as a Bear	78	Deborah	A bee, to speak kind words
79	Sebastian	Revered	79	Betty	God's oath
80	Ernest	Earnest, Sincere	80	Anastasia	Resurrection
81	Gary	Spear carrier	81	Erica	Ever Powerful Ruler
82	Gregory	Vigilant, Watchful	82	Haley	Hero

83	Larry	Crowned with Laurel	83	Whitney	From the white island
84	Andrew	Courageous, Valiant, Man	84	Pamela	Honeyed
85	Joseph	God Will Increase	85	Vivian	Lively
86	Robert	Bright, Famous	86	Jane	God is Gracious
87	Cody	Assistant, a cushion, possessions	87	Dominique	Belonging to God
88	Patrick	Noble	88	Rebecca	Bound, tied
89	Jeffrey	Peace of God	89	Candace	White-hot, glowing, glittering
90	Jared	One who rules	90	Abby	Head of a monastery
91	Dustin	Valiant fighter, dark stone	91	Joy	Joy
92	Trevor	Cautious	92	Sonia	Wisdom
93	Edward	Guardian of prosperity, guardian of the mists	93	Tyler	Tiler, roofer
94	Antonio	Flower	94	Macy	From Matthew's land, club
95	Seth	Appointed	95	Frances	Of France
96	Spencer	Dispenser	96	Demy	Half, small
97	George	Farmer	97	Loraine	Gracious Laurel
98	Raymond	Worthy protector	98	Astrid	Star, super strength, divine strength
99	Oscar	Divine spear	99	Sophie	Wisdom
100	Philip	Horses lover	100	Cassidy	Clever

Top 20 Sexy Girl Names with Analysis

1. Emma – The name of Emma creates a restless, creative nature that takes you into many ventures. Yours is a versatile, musical, artistic, but independent nature and you must have the freedom to express your creative ideas and abilities to be happy. This name also gives you a love of home and family, and as a parent, you would likely be fair and understanding.

2. Jessica – Your name of Jessica has given you a responsible, expressive, inspirational and friendly personality. Self-confidence has made it easy for you to meet people and you are well-liked for yours spontaneous, happy ways. You sincerely like people and do not often experience loneliness.

3. Christine – As Christine you seek change, travel new opportunities, and new challenges. Your active, restless nature demands action and you dislike system and monotony. As you are versatile and capable, you could do any job well, although you would not like to do menial tasks. You are not afraid to risk a gamble as the name gives you much self-confidence.

4. Michelle – Your name of Michelle has made you a hard worker with a meticulous sense of detail. You have a great deal of patience and independence, and you can be relied upon to complete your undertakings. You are stable, trustworthy and home loving. You resist change.

5. Ashley – Your name of Ashley has given you a rather quiet, reserved, serious, studious nature. You have sensitivity and appreciation for the finer and deeper things of life, the beauties of nature, music, art and literature. The people who mean the most to you are those who can offer you intellectual companionship.

6. Nicole – The name of Nicole has created a congenial nature with the desire to associate in friendship and understanding both socially and in the business world. You have a clever, quick mind, with the ability to accomplish a great deal in a short period of time, although it is not easy for you to systematize your efforts.

7. Jennifer – The name of Jennifer leads you to assume considerable responsibility and to prefer to work independently, without direction or interference from other because you have very definite ideas of your own. This name does make you quite direct and straight –to-the-point.

8. Victoria – The name of Victoria has given you a quick-minded, sensitive nature. It gives you a clever, creative ability in art, music, singing or drama and an appreciation for refined surroundings. As you respond to love and encouragement from others, your romantic and dreamy nature can easily lead you into love affairs.

9. Angelina – Your name of Angelina has made you versatile and creative. There is hardly anything you cannot do if you put your mind to it but a driving urge leads you to one experience after another, seldom finishing what you start. As soon as a challenge is met, boredom sets in, and you yearn for another experience.

10. Carmen – Your name of Carmen makes you very idealistic and generous. You want to assume responsibilities and to look after people, however, you can become too involved in other people's problems and tend to worry. You desire a settled home and family life, and are expressive and attentive to your loved ones.

11. Samantha – Your name of Samantha has given you the desire for the best that money can buy: good clothes, and refined surroundings, all the finer things of life, although you might be inclined to get things through the influence of others rather than through hard work. You always strive to create a good impression.

12. Natalie – Your name of Natalie has given you a desire for self-expression and for positions that allow contact with people, free from the restrictions and monotony into which you are often drawn. You strive to different and have the self-confidence to implement your ideas because you have the perseverance necessary to see something through, despite obstacles. Although you meet new people easily, it is not easy to you to maintain a relaxed, harmonious relationship.

13. Stephanie – Your name of Stephanie contributes sensitive, creative and idealistic qualities to your nature that could be expressed in a variety of literary or artistic fields. Although mentally quick and intuitive, you experience a lack of fluency in verbal expression in responding. Your emotional feelings are easily affected and you will be always involved in other people's problems as a result of your overly sympathetic nature.

14. Sydney – The name of Sydney creates a very versatile and creative nature. You are quick-minded and have the freedom of expression to mix easily with people. You seek change in order to have the opportunity for travel, new experiences, and new friends and associates. As you are naturally talkative, you find it easy to meet and make friends with many people. This name inclines you to be sympathetic and generous to those in difficult and unfortunate circumstances.

15. Naomi – As Naomi you have a great love of nature and the out-of-doors. All the finer things of life and beauties of nature are an inspiration to you and you are attracted to the mysteries of nature. The average person would never realize the true depth of your nature.

16. Kimberly -The name Kimberly gives you a strongly independent and highly creative nature, with drive and ambition to have experiences and accomplish things out of the ordinary.You are friendly, sociable and charming person. While you find it easy to meet and mix, and can appear agreeable and compromising in conversation, you can become unbending and forceful if pressed too far.

17. Vanessa - Your first name of Vanessa has created a deep, sensitive, refined nature with an intelligent mind. You can be lifted by beauty in all forms and are at the most creative when inspired. Your expressive, affectionate nature responds quickly through your feelings, but you must guard against being possessive and jealous.

18. Lindsay - Your name of Lindsay creates a desire for association with people and new experiences. This name has given you a gregarious personality and a quick-thinking, creative, and versatile nature, but one that is very emotional. You like to make your own decisions and to be the master of your domain. You feel a limitation in your own expression when it is necessary to reach another through tact and understanding.

19. Chantel -Your name of Chantel makes you very idealistic and generous, with the strong desire to uplift humanity leading you into situations where you can express your desire to serve others. You have a serious desire to understand the heart and mind of everyone, and could be very effective in a career or in volunteer work where you are handling people and serving in a humanitarian way.

20. Elizabeth – The name of Elizabeth gives you leadership qualities and you are seldom happy in positions where you must direction from others. Material and financial success are the focus of your interests. You have a very independent, practical, analytical nature with skillful business abilities. Whatever you undertake, you have the patience and determination to do well. Difficulty in accepting advice or admitting that you may have made a mistake causes you to appear to be stubborn and set in your ways.

Top 20 Sexy Boy Names with Analysis

1. Michael – *Your name of Michael has given you very practical hard-working, systematic nature. You have a clever mind, a sense of responsibility, good business judgment, and an appreciation of the finer things of life. You are serious minded and in your younger years you have more mature interests than other your age.*

2. William – *The name of William gives you very individual, reserved, serious nature. You prefer to be alone with your own thoughts, rather than in the company of others. Home and family mean a great deal to you and it is natural that you should desire the security of a peaceful, settled home environment.*

3. Christopher – *The name of Christopher incorporates a potential aptitude for concentration and patient, logical thought along mechanical or scientific lines. You gravitate to situations where you have stability and the opportunity to make slow step by step progress. This name creates a deliberate and methodical way of thinking and speaking; it takes you time to learn but, once you have mastered a subject, you do not forget it.*

4. Matthew – *The name of Matthew gives you a generous quality to your nature. This name causes you to be somewhat too concerned with the personalities, problems, and activities of other people, but you must guard carefully against giving more than you receive or you will find yourself doing without because you have helped someone else.*

5. Kyle – *The name of Kyle creates a very aggressive and independent nature, one with big ambitions, giving you original, progressive, large-scale ideas, salesmanship and promotional ability as well as the excellent business judgment, which enables you to gain the financial accumulation to which you feel entitled.*

6. Jason – *The name of Jason has given you the desire to meet and mix socially and to create congenial circumstances for everyone. You are good at sales work and you could do well because of your friendly personality, interest in people, and desire to please. Your ideas can be very original and inventive.*

7. Brad – *The name of Brad has made you serious-minded, responsible, and stable. You love the security of a home and family, you are fond of children, and, as a parent you would be fair and understanding. You have a diplomatic and tactful manner and possess a charming, easy-going nature which puts people at ease. People are drawn to you because they feel that you are patient, kind, understanding, and responsive.*

8. Daniel - As Daniel you have a great love of nature and the out-of-doors, and could have a desire to be in an occupation, which takes you outdoors and involves you with the products of the earth. You are not overly ambitious, preferring instead to seek stable, settled conditions which are adequate to meet your responsibilities. You like to be your own boss and you are capable of handling responsibilities for others.

9. Joey – The name of Joey has given you a very imaginative, creative mind. You always have new ideas, but too often, they are for an easy way out of a difficulty, or an easy way of making money. You seek change in order to have the opportunity for travel, new experiences, and new friends and associates. You desire independence and freedom from the authority and interference of others.

10. Joshua – Your name of Joshua gives you the ability to be creative along practical lines and endeavor. Your personal appearance is important to you, for you desire to make a good impression on others. Your pleasant manner attracts people to you with their problems and you are capable of offering practical advice, though you would probably not follow such advice yourself.

11. David – Your first name of David has given you a very systematic nature .In reaching your goals, you are very independent and resourceful, patient and determined. You can be very positive and definite in your own ideas and opinions. Also, this name does not incorporate qualities that enable you to be diplomatic and to compromise.

12. Dylan – The name of Dylan creates a very passive, easy-going, friendly nature. You love people and desire to get along with everyone you meet. Your creative nature and ambition drive you to pursue success to the extent that you jeopardize your personal well-being. People are drawn to you because they feel that you are patient, kind, understanding, and responsive.

13. Ryan – The name of Ryan has created a most expressive nature, idealistic and inspirational, driven a strong inner urge to be of service in some way that would up lift humanity. You would be successful in any position dealing with the public as you have a diplomatic and tactful manner and possess a charming, easy-going nature which puts people at ease. You love the security of a home and family.

14. Nick - Your first name of Nick makes you extremely generous. You have a bubbling, spontaneous nature and a happy-go-lucky outlook which helps smooth the pathway of life. Also you are sympathetic to the needs of others. Your spontaneous expression stands you in good stead during arguments or debates.You are fun and party loving person.

15. Paul - Your name of Paul gives you self-assurance, independence, and confidence. You have depth of mind and the ability to concentrate and to follow a line of thought to a logical conclusion. Your love of challenging the concepts of others invariably leads you to create your own ideas and to pioneer new lines of thought. Your strong characteristic of individuality qualifies you as a leader.

16. Justin - Your name of Leo makes you quick-minded, versatile, and very expressive. You have the ability to create a favourable first impression, and so you could do well in the fields of sales promotion or entertainment. You are adaptable and creative in responding to new situations. You like to finish what you start without interruptions, and also to have everything in its place and properly organized.

17. Jacob - The name of Jacob creates a quiet, systematic, and technical nature and a clever, inventive mind, attentive to detail. You are attracted to working outdoors in nature, where you would experience the peace and serenity you so much desire. You are inclined to be quiet, reserved, patient, and conservative, preferring to test and prove everything to your own satisfaction before committing yourself.

18. Anthony - Your first name of Anthony has given you an expressive, diplomatic, and gracious nature. You have a good appreciation of material values, business ability, and skill in organizing and managing others. You have very expensive tastes, and your desires could well exceed your initiative in providing for them through your own efforts. Personal appearance is important to you. You are always well-groomed yourself, and you judge others by your own standard.

19. James - While your name of James gives you an intense desire to be of service to others, it brings out a practical, technical nature, and you become involved in fussy little details that detract from the fulfilment of your greater ideals. You are a very patient person and will work hard one step at a time to accomplish your goals. Not interested in large undertakings, you are content to live from day to day to save for your future. Always budgeting carefully, you do not believe in frivolous spending.

20. Max - The name of Max creates a very aggressive and independent nature, one with big ambitions, giving you original, progressive, large-scale ideas, salesmanship and promotional ability as well as the excellent business judgment, which enables you to gain the financial accumulation to which you feel entitled. You are seldom satisfied and are always seeking something new. You like to be your own boss and you are capable of handling responsibilities for others.

Name Teams

Names with "Strong" Meanings

Abd-Al-Aziz	Servant of the Powerful	Arabic(m)
Abdul	Servant	Arabic(m)
Alcippe	Mighty Mare	Latin(f)
Aziz	Powerful, Great	Arabic (m)
Berk	Firm, Steadfast	Turkish(m)
Carlisle	Strong as the Shining One	Old English(m)
Gabriel	Strength of God	Hebrew(m)
Ikaika	Strong	Hawaiian(m)
Iphigenia	Mythical Creature	Greek(f)
Jelani	Powerful Might	African(m)
Jirair	Strong, Hardworking	Armenian(m)
Ken	Helmeted chief	Gaelic(m)
Kenji	Strong, Healthy Second Son	Japanese(m)
Magnhild	Powerful Battle	Norwegian(f)
Metin	Strong	Turkish(m)
Valentine	Good health	Latin(m)
Valerius	Strength, Valor	Ancient Roman(m)
Waltraud	Rule strength	Teutonic(f)

Names with "Brave" Meanings

Archibald	Bold Prince	Anglo-Saxon(m)
Baldric	Bold, Powerful, Brave Ruler	Old English(m)
Baldwin	Brave Friend	German(m)
Bernard	Bold as a Bear	German(m)
Burkhard	Brave Protector	German(m)
Eckhard	Brave Swordsman	German(m)
Everard	Brave Boar	Old English(m)
Gebhard	Brave Gift	German(m)
Gerard	Spear, Brave	Old German(m)
Giffard	Brave Gift	Old English(m)
Hartmann	Brave Man	German(m)
Hartmut	Brave Mind	German(m)
Howard	Guardian of the home,watchman	English(m)
Kenelm	Brave Helmet	Old English(m)
Leonard	Lion-hearted	Old German(m)
Nanna	Graceful one	Hebrew(f)
Wyatt	Little warrior,water	Old English(m)

Names with "Intelligent" Meanings

Albert	Noble, Bright	German(m)
Bert	Fortress	Old English(m)
Bertram	Bright	German(m)
Berthold	Glorious ruler	Teutonic(m)
Bertha	Brilliant, Illuminated Fame	German(f)
Bilge	Wise	Turkish(f)
Clara	Clear, Illuminated	Latin(f)
Clarice	Clear, Illuminated	French(f)
Colbert	Cool, Bright	Old English(m)
Cuthbert	Bright Fame	Old English(m)
Delbert	Bright Valley	Old English(m)
Eirian	Illuminating Beauty	Welsh(f)
Engelbert	Bright as an Angel	German(m)
Frode	Wisdom	Danish(m)
Gilbert	Bright Pledge	Dutch(m)
Gladwyn	Bright Friend	Old English(m)
Herbert	Bright Army Ruler	French(m)
Hubert	Brilliant Heart and Mind	Dutch(m)
Kalea	Bright, Clear	Hawaiian(f)
Kunibert	Brave, Bright	German(m)
Lambert	Wealthy in land	Latin(m)
Leocadia	Clear, Shining	Spanish(f)
Noga	Bright	Hebrew(f)
Norbert	Blonde hero	German(m)
Robert	Bright,famous	Old English(m)
Savio	Intelligent	Italian(m)
Shannon	Wise, River	Irish(f)
Shirley	Bright Meadow	Old English(f&m)
Sumati	Wisdom	Hindu(f&m)
Ziv	Very bright	Hebrew(f&m)

Names with "Happy" Meanings

Abigel	God is Joy	Modern English(f)
Aasher	Blessed, Happy	Modern English(m)
Aliza	Joyful	Hebrew(f)
Fortunato	Fortunate	Italian(m)
Freyde	Joy	Yiddish(f)
Gay	Happy	Old English(f)
Gilah	Joyful	Hebrew(f)
Gioconda	Joyful	Italian(f)
Happy	Joyful	English(f&m)
Joy	Joy	Old English(f)
Letitia	Joy, Gladness	Latin(f)
Liron	Joyful Song	Hebrew(m&f)
Meriwether	Merry Weather	Middle English(m&f)
Rada	Joyful	Czechoslovakian(f)
Radomil	Joyful, Favored	Bulgarian(m)
Simcha	Joyful	Hebrew(f&m)
Winston	Joy Stone	Old English(m)

Names with "Beautiful" Meanings

Alana	Attractive	Gaelic(f)
Anwen	Stunningly Beautiful	Welsh(f)
Aoibheann	Beautiful Patina	Gaelic(f)
Beau	Beautiful, Handsome	French(m)
Beaumont	Beautiful Mountain	French(m)
Beauregard	Beautiful, Handsome View	French(m)
Bellanita	Gracious Beauty	French(f)
Belle	Beautiful	French(f)
Branwen	White, Fair, Blessed Hill	Welsh(f)
Calanthe	Beautiful Flower	Old English(f)
Calogero	Elderly Beauty	Italian(m)
Caoimhe	Beautiful	Celtic(f)
Coinneach	Handsome	Gaelic(m)
Erianthe	Sweet as Many Flowers	Greek(f)
Grazyna	Beautiful	Lithuanian(f)
Graziella	Graceful Beauty	Italian(f)
Isolde	Beautiful	Celtic(f)
Jaffe	Beauty	Hebrew(f)
Jamil	Attractive	Arabic(m)
Keefe	Handsome, Beloved	Gaelic(m)
Kevin	Handsome, Gentle, Beloved	Gaelic(f)
Linda	Beautiful	Spanish(f)
Mabelle	Lovable, Beautiful	Old English(f)
MacKenzie	Son of the wise leader	Gaelic(m&f)
Nava	Beauty	Hebrew(f)
Rosabella	Beautiful Rose	Italian(f)
Sigrid	Winning adviser	Old Norse(f)
Zuri	Attractive	African(f)

Names with "Lucky" Meanings

Felix	Happy	Latin(m)
Fortunato	Fortunate	Italian(m)
Fortune	Fortunate	Old English(f)
Madoc	Blessed	Welsh(m)
Prosper	Prosperous, Successful	French(m)
Shreya	Auspicious	Hindu(f)
Xiang	Fragrant Flight	Chinese(m&f)

Names with "Generous" Meanings

Aimo	Generous	Finnish(m)
Charity	Charity, Kind	Latin(f)
Ithel	Generous Prince	Welsh(m)
Karim	Giving, Noble	Arabic(m)
Theodosius	Gift of God	Greek(m)

Names with "Royal" Meanings

Abd-Al-Malik	Servant of the King	Arabic(m)
Almira	Princess	Old English(f)
Armel	Prince	French(m)
Basil	Royal, Brave	Greek(m)
Donald	World Leader	Old English(m)
Edric	Blessed, Powerful Ruler	Old English(m)
Elric	Elf Ruler	Old English(m)
Emyr	King	Welsh(m)
Eric	Ever Powerful Ruler	Scandinavian(m)
Fitzroy	Son of the King	Old English(m)
Frederick	Peaceful, Powerful Ruler	Old English(m)
Friedhold	Peaceful Ruler	German(m)
Gruffydd	Prince	Welsh(m)
Harold	Army Ruler	Old English(m)
Henry	Ruler of the Home	Old English(m)
Idris	Enthusiastic Prince	Welsh(m)
Ithel	Generous Prince	Welsh(m)
Lareyna	Queen	Spanish(f)
Leroy	King	Old French(m)
Reagan	Little King	Gaelic(m&f)
Regina	Queen	Latin(f)
Reine	Queen	Latin(f)
Rex	King	Latin(m)
Rhiannon	A mythological nymph	Welsh(f)
Rhodri	King Wheel	Welsh(m)
Roald	Fame power	Teutonic(m)
Ryan	Little King	Gaelic(m&f)
Sarah	Princess	Hebrew(f)
Torvald	Thor's Ruler	Scandinavian(m)
Walter	Army Ruler	Old German(m)
Xerxes	Prince	Persian(m)
Zoltan	Life, Sultan	Hungarian(m)

Names with "Religious" Meanings

Abd-Allah	Servant of God	Arabic(m)
Abiel	God is My Father	Hebrew(m)
Abijah	Yahweh is My God	Hebrew(m)
Abimael	God is My Father	Hebrew(m)
Adalia	Yahweh is Just	Hebrew(m)
Adonai	My Lord	Hebrew(m)
Adonijah	Lord is Yahweh	Hebrew(m)
Amariah	Yahweh Has Spoken	Hebrew(m)
Ammiel	My Kinsman is God	Hebrew(m)
Anselm	Divine Protection	Old English(m)
Ansgar	Spear god	German(m)
Ariel	Lion of God	Hebrew(m&f)
Asbjorn	Bear god	Norwegian(m)
Azarel	Helped by God	Hebrew(m)
Beelzebub	Fly Lord	Hebrew(m)
Benaiah	Yahweh has Created	Hebrew(m)
Bethel	House of God	Hebrew(f)
Bethuel	Man of God	Hebrew(m)
Bithiah	Yahweh's Daughter	Hebrew(f)
Bogumil	God's Favor	Polish(m)
Boguslaw	Glory of God	Polish(m)
Bohumir	God is Peaceful	Czechoslovakian(m)
Cedric	Lord of Wars	Old English(m)
Chibuzo	God Leads	African(m&f)
Cyriacus	Of the Lord	Ancient Roman(m)
Cyril	Lord	Old English(m)
Daniel	God is My Judge	Old English(m)
Delaiah	Drawn by Yahweh	Hebrew(m)
Devdan	Gift of God	Hindu(m)
Dominic	Belonging to God	Old English(m)

Dorothea	Gift of God	Dutch(f)
Eliezer	God is My Helper	Hebrew(m)
Elihu	Yahweh is God	Hebrew(m)
Elijah	The Lord is My God	Old English(m)
Elizabeth	Consecrated to God	Old English(f)
Elkanah	Created by God	Hebrew(m)
Emmanuel	God is With Us	Hebrew(m)
Gabriel	Strength of God	French(m)
Geoffrey	Peace of God	Old English(m)
Goddard	Brave god	Old English(m)
Godelieve	God's Love	Dutch(m)
Godfrey	Peace of God	Old English(m)
Godiva	Gift of God	Old English(f)
Godwin	Friend of God	Old English(m)
Gotthold	God's Love	German(m)
Hananiah	Yahweh is Gracious	Hebrew(m)
Hazael	Sees God	Hebrew(m)
Ishmael	God Will Hear	Old English(m)
Israel	Wrestles With God	Hebrew(m)
Jessica	God Watches	Old English(f)
Jonathan	God Has Given	Old English(m)
Joshua	God Saves	Old English(m)
Mathew	Gift of God	Old English(m)
Osborn	Divine, Bear	Old English(m)
Raphael	God Has Healed	French(m)
Theodore	Gift of God	French(m)
Timothy	To Honor God	Old English(m)
Zechariah	Remembered by God	Old English(m)

Names with "Flowery" Meanings

Anthony	Flower	Old English(m)
Blodeuyn	Blossom	Welsh(f)
Blossom	Flower bud	Old English(f)
Bluma	Flower	Hebrew(f)
Calanthe	Beautiful Flower	Old English(f)
Fioralba	Flower at Dawn	Italian(f)
Fiorella	Flower	Italian(f)
Fiorenza	Flourishing, Blooming, Prosperous	Italian(f)
Floriana	Gracious Flower	Italian(f)
Flower	Flower	Old English(f)
Iolanthe	Violet Flower	Old English(f)
Ornella	Blooming Ash Tree	Italian(f)
Rhosyn	Rose	Welsh(f)
Rosa	Rose	Latin(f)
Rosabella	Beautiful Rose	Italian(f)
Rosalia	Rose	Italian(f)
Rosalinda	Beautiful Rose	English(f)
Rosalyn	Beautiful Rose	Old English(f)
Rosamunda	Pure Rose	Latin(f)
Susanna	Lily	Old English(f)
Zahrah	Blooming Flower	Arabic(f)

Names with "Elfin" Meanings

Alfhild	Elf Battle	Norwegian(f)
Alfredia	Elf Counselor	Modern English(f)
Alfihar	Elf Army	German(m)
Alger	Elf Spear	Old Greman(m)
Alvin	Elf Friend	Old English(m)
Auberon	Noble, Elf Bear	Old English(m)
Aubrey	Elf Power	Old English(m&f)
Elric	Elf Ruler	Old English(m)
Elwood	Elf Wood	Old English(m)
Siofra	Elf	Irish(f)

Female names associated with "Flowers"

Amaryllis	Fresh and Sparkling Flower	Old English
Anemone	Wind Flower	Greek
April	4h Month, Blossoming	Latin
Camellia	Floweing Shrub	Old English
Celandine	Celandine Flower	Old English
Chrysanta	Chrysanthemum	Old English
Clover	Clover Flower	Old English
Daffodil	Daffodil Flower	Old English
Dahlia	Flower Named for Botanist A. Dahl	Hebrew
Daisy	Daisy Flower	Old English
Eglantine	Sweetbrier Flower	Old English
Flora	Flower	Latin
Gardenia	Tropical Flower	Old English
Heather	Flowering Shrub	Old English
Iris	Iris Flower	Greek
Ivy	Vine	Greek
Jasmine	Jasmine, Fragrant Flower	Persian
Lavender	Flower, Light Purple Color	Old English
Lily	Lily Flower	Latin
Linnea	Lime tree, national flower of Sweden	Norwegian
Lotus	Lotus Flower	Greek
Magnolia	Flower	French
Marigold	Golden Flower	Greek
Narcissa	Narcissus	Greek
Pansy	Pansy Flower	Old English
Petunia	Petunia Flower	Latin
Primrose	Primrose Flower, meaning First Rose	Old English
Rose	Rose	French
Violet	Violet Flower	Latin
Zinnia	Zinnia Flower	Old English

Numerology and the Destiny Baby Number

It is time to reveal the secrets of your baby name using numerology! Probably, you have already chosen some baby names. Select one baby name and write it down. Now assign numbers to each letter using the chart below. The chart is read downwards so that 1 is A, J, S; 2 is B, K, T; etc.

Number Assignments

1	2	3	4	5	6	7	8	9
A	B	C	D	E	F	G	H	I
J	K	L	M	N	O	P	Q	R
S	T	U	V	W	X	Y	Z	-

For example, I will use Amanda as a baby name. Now I assign numerical values to Amanda's full name using the chart.

AMANDA – 1+4+1+5+4+1

Now add all numbers together:

AMANDA = 16 or (7)

In numerology, 16 become 7 (1+6). Most two-digit numbers get "broken down" in the same way. The only exceptions are the "master numbers" (11, 22). When a master number appears in the final total, it can be read two ways (11=2 and 22=4) or (11, 22).

As you can see from the above calculations, Amanda's name reduces to a 7. In numerology, this particular combination provides the "Destiny Number".

Let's check what Amanda's destiny number is! After that, choose a baby name and find its secrets!

On the chart below is a quick interpretation of the numbers 1 through 9 and the two master numbers 11 and 22. Enjoy!

The Numbers Revealed!	
1	is ambitious, independent, self-confident,. money-oriented, decisive, and stern.
2	is supportive, diplomatic, analytical, responsible, careful, and domestic..
3	is enthusiastic, optimistic, fun-loving, friendly, vigorous and holiday-maker.
4	is practical, traditional, serious, spiritual, eccentric, and a bit of a loner.
5	is adventurous, mercurial, sensual, good-hearted, powerful and fashionable.
6	is kind-hearted, industrious, creative, well-bred, tenacious and sensitive.
7	is clever, quick-minded, creative, curious, jealous and mysterious.
8	is expressive, generous, artsy-craftsy, tactful, conversable and self-opinionated.
9	is multi-talented, compassionate, global, t, athletic, stubborn and selfish.
11	is enlightened, intense, high-strung, intuitive, smart and vindictive. (Also read the "lower" vibration of 2 above.)
22	is goal-oriented, a global planner, inspired,good humoured, and sociable. (Also read the "lower" vibration of 4 above.)

Numerology and Lucky Rich Baby Names

This time, numerology implies wealthy and not wealthy numbers. If the numbers in the following chart are with "$", they are the lucky rich numbers. This means, that if your baby name has "$" numbers, she or he will be fortunate and well-to-do in life!

1$	2	**3$**	4	**5$**	**6$**	**7$**	**8$**	9	10
11$	12	**13$**	14	**15$**	**16$**	**17$**	**18$**	19	20
21$	22	**23$**	**24$**	**25$**	26	27	28	**29$**	30
31$	**32$**	**33$**	34	**35$**	36	**37$**	38*	**39$**	40
41$	42	43	44	**45$**	46	**47$**	**48$**	49	50
51*	**52$**	53	54	55*	56	**57$**	58*	59	60
61*	62	**63$**	64	**65$**	66	**67$**	**68$**	69	70
71*	72*	**73$**	74	75*	76	77*	78*	79	80
81$									

Note! The numbers with "*" are extremely clever numbers. This means, that if your baby name has "*", the baby will be genius! All the other numbers are good-natured numbers, which means that your baby will be very good-hearted and sensitive!

To apply on baby name, I count how many letters in the name to determine if the name is lucky rich name or not. For example, I choose the name David Franklin Peterson.

	FIRST NAME	MIDDLE NAME	LAST NAME
FULL NAME	DAVID	FRANKLIN	PETERSON
LETTER COUNT	5	8	8

You can see that 5, 8 and 8 are Lucky Rich Numbers!

Now choose a baby name and check if it is Lucky Rich Name! ☺

Five Fun Facts about Names

1. *Every child has an official right to have a name.* Article 24-3 of the U.N. International Covenant on Civil and Political Rights says so. Why was this declaration necessary? The U.N. recognized that children born into war zones, extreme poverty, and refugee camps may not have their births registered, making them especially vulnerable to all kinds of abuse.

2. *The U.S. Census Bureau estimates that 88,000 different last names account for more than 90 percent of the 280 million people in the U.S.* By contrast, China--with its population of more than 1 billion--has only 150 to 400 basic surnames. Clear proof of the diversity of America's melting-pot society.

3. *When it comes to variety in names, girls rule.* Again, according to the Census Bureau, approximately 90 percent of the U.S. population is covered by 4,275 different girls' names, but only 1,219 different boys' names. Why so many fewer names for boys than for girls? It may be that boys' names are more tradition-bound, because boys are more likely to be named after a relative. Another possibility: Although this is changing, our society still clings to the assumption that boys will eventually have to get "serious" jobs (and so need serious-sounding names), while girls won't, leaving more leeway for creativity, if not frivolity.

4. *Anemonyms (a truly lovely word) are the names of winds and storms.* Once a name has been associated with a violent hurricane, that name is retired. There will never be another Hurricane Hugo, for instance. The Weather Service also tries to pick names that are easy to pronounce and culturally sensitive.

5. *Toponyms are place names.* Early U.S. names mirrored places in the old country (New England, for example), honored English royalty (Virginia, after Queen Elizabeth, known as the Virgin Queen), or celebrated the Pilgrims' survival (Providence). America itself, however, was named after Italian navigator and explorer Amerigo Vespucci in the early 16th century.

ASTROLOGY
Names for Every Month

January

January people are patient and reserved. They endure all the troubles with stoicism, and they share their inmost with difficulty even with those who are closest to them. January women are with a firm, man's character, secretive and independent. They are proud and highly appreciate their independence. Family life with them is not easy because of their permanent aspiration after leadership, but they are devoted wives and are always ready to support their husbands. At that, women are expert cooks, but they don't like cleaning and do it perforce. January men are courageous and just people, they can be relied on in a difficult moment. They are decisive in their deeds, they often behave without considering those around them and they are inclined to unjustified risk. They are patronizing to people weaker than they are, they treat women with respect and they are capable of forgiving everything. They are proud and possess strong will. They are wonderful husbands. January children should have names with soft sounding aimed at neutralizing the excessive hardness of their nature and softening their pride. Appropriate names are: Ashley, Melanie, Holly, Wendy, Selena, Matthew, Anthony, Kyle, Samuel, Lucas.

February

February people are persistent, persevering and too unbalanced, though unlike December ones they are capable of exercising control over themselves. Their nature is complicated, unpredictable, they are subjected to nervous collapses. They are very courageous and are not afraid of difficulties. They make decisions fast, indeed, they are sometimes incorrect.Unlike January people they forgive insults with difficulty, some of them are rancorous and revengeful. They are not inclined to play noble and magnanimous, they despise the weak. They are too straightforward and egoistical. By nature they are careerists, they are capable of not particularly plausible deeds aimed at attaining their objectives, they know how to manipulate people. It is inherent for them that they go from one extreme to the other. They like children and there are often more children in their families. Appropriate names are: Sebastian, Oliver, Robert, Edward, James, Rebecca, Astrid, Deborah, Courtney, Sandra.

March

March people are very sensitive and susceptible. They endure failure with difficulty and this is why they slowly climb up the official ladder. Although they show obstinacy and persistence, this is often to their detriment. They are cowardly, indecisive, easily vulnerable. They consider that they do not go well on in life. It is not in vain that there are many ill-fated and envious persons amongst March people. They strive after success all their lives but they remain unrecognized. If they manage to climb to the top of the glory in spite of that, this is usually not for long and falling down from there means collapse of all their hopes for them. Such allegedly spring people are self-centered and ambitious. They are irritable, waspish, and accept other people's successes as their own defeat. They are phlegmatic and heap up the people close to them with their endless complaints from fate. They are mistrustful, they believe in prejudice and they often turn to fortune-tellers. Men are grumbles, they are difficult to please and excessively squeamish. Women waste a lot of time for their dressing, they pay great attention to their appearance, they stay in front of the mirror for hours on end before leaving home. Such children had better be given names with hard sounding to add more decisiveness, tenacity to their nature so that the child could feel more confident in him or herself. Appropriate names are: Hillary, Virginia, Monica, Marta, Veronica, Aron, Scott, George, Trevor, Roland.

April

April people possess a firmer nature than March ones. They persistently pursue their goals, they are brave and decisive, regardless of the fact that they do not always succeed in realizing themselves adequately. They are practical and sober-minded. They are most excited in the material side of life. They are easily promoted in their jobs and they know what they want. They have enough luck but they are superfluously ambitious. In marriage, they rely more on reason than on feelings. They give up their ordinary way of life with difficulty. Stability and material welfare are the most important for men. They would rather agree to endure wives they do not love than destroy their marriage replacing material welfare with love. Women born in April, however, have different attitude to family life. They appreciate good relations with their husbands, the material side remaining for them in the background. April women are cheerful, witty, and they may find out a reason for merriment in each trifle. Those born in April had better be given names as: Victoria, Andrea, Britney, Kylie, Whitney, Ernest, Andrew, Philip, Oscar, Jonathan.

May

May people are people of principles and uncompromising, domineering and fussy. They may instantly discontinue their relationship and they get easily divorced, though they regret it after that. It is difficult to create a solid family with women born in May, they strive for leadership positions, and they do not endure objections. They are interested in material prosperity most of all, and in events of bad relationships with their husbands, they easily find entertainments beyond their family. Men born in May are good husbands, they manage to provide for their families and to obtain the right to be respected. Although with firm nature, they are more yielding in their family than out of it. They are greatly influenced by women's tears, complaints, failures. They are always ready to help the fair sex, and this is why they often find themselves in awkward situations. Babies born in May should have names as: Erica, Haley, Sonia, Tyler, Sophie, Spencer, Antonio, Patrick, Larry, Kelvin.

June

June people are very vulnerable, mistrustful. They are cautious in their deeds, sometimes overplaying safe. They are good and compassionate, but too pigeon-hearted to struggle with anyone. They have many talents by nature, they are practical and enterprising. They are often turned to for advice and moral support. They show their emotions with people close to them rather reservedly, but they may be more open with people, whom they do not know so well. They avoid conflicts, at the June men are a little cowardly and weak-willed, when the matter is about personal problems. On that account they are lucky professionally, they are happy in love, in the interest of the truth often out of their family. Amorous by nature, they are easily carried away but not for long. They do not bear moral admonitions and they themselves do not like to preach to people. They are very clean, some of them up to squeamishness. Women know how to create comfort at home and men do their best so that the family would not suffer material difficulties. Appropriate names are: Leslie, Brandy, Lauren, Larissa, Valentine, Frank, Dennis, Jimmy, Simon, Martin.

July

Unstable nervous system, impatience, egotism, irritability - these are the characteristic features of July people. They are proud and independent. Egotists. Weak-willed, they may not refuse anything to their friends and they become drunks easily (this refers to men most of all). Women strive for leadership, they try to command their husbands, they often complain to their relatives and friends of their fate, they openly tell them about the confusion in their families. It is difficult to please them, they are always dissatisfied with something. Men are quite good-natured, carefree, they often make mistakes. As far as women are concerned, they are credulous and naive. If they are deceived once in their feelings, they become confirmed bachelorettes. They endure all troubles in silence, and they do not like to complain of their fate. They may unburden their hearts solely to their mothers, since their mothers are the persons closest to them by soul. Appropriate names are: Judy, Eva, Helen, Mary and Dennis.

August

Too emotional, energetic, persevering. Purposeful in their actions, but not cautious. They do not stand phlegmatic people, who irritate them. August women are confident of their strength, they are not rancorous but they are distrustful. They are leaders in their families. They are good homemakers, but they do not enjoy cooking a lot. Men are sensitive by nature, and they are yielding in their family relationships. They are seldom happy in their first marriage. They do not stand pressure and criticism, they are irritable and expect solely praise and universal acknowledgement. They are very jealous, although they themselves are seldom faithful spouses. They are vulnerable and like children, they require enhanced attention to them from those surrounding them. Appropriate names are: Stacy, Cindy, Caroline, Sabrina, Racheal, Bobby, Markus, Greg, John.

September

Quick-tempered, emotional, purposeful people. They like giving presents, but otherwise not too generous, they would not spend a cent in vain. They try to look open-handed in the eyes of the people surrounding them but they rarely do it without considering their personal interests first. They are calculating and self-centered. Women worry most about themselves than about their husbands, men do not know how to provide for their families, but they will never injure their own feelings. They do not regret losing a great sum of money but if their wives buy expensive garments without their knowledge, they will reproach them of wasting too much money. September people enjoy the company of their friends, but they will never skip their personal benefit even if this is to the detriment of their closest friends. They refund their debts with difficulty and they often forget about them. They do not endure scenes of jealousy, in such events they behave out of spite. They are very jealous themselves. Women are impatient and very independent. They like to sleep until late in the morning and they are often late for work, turning this into something normal. Otherwise, they are wonderful homemakers and everything shines at their homes. They enjoy cooking and are able to cook delicious dishes.

Men are too cautious, things come to the contraction of a marriage. Appropriate names are: names are: Kristen, Marissa, Daniel, Julia, Shannon, Mark, Steven, Paul, Peter, Thomas.

October

They are strict, but solely in the events when this refers to their work. They think that it is not always obligatory to be such with their friends. They like to tell fibs and they are witty and enterprising. They are unselfish in the relations with their friends but they are practical and careful in financial operations. They are magnanimous. They do not hurry to draw conclusions and they do not make any rash decisions. They try to listen to as many options as possible, on whose grounds they build up their very close people being of authority for them. Women are objective persons of principles. They have a good memory and easily build up their careers. They do not forgive treasons and betrayal. They try to preserve their families with all their might, where they are leaders and they rarely lean on their on their husbands. Men are practical, sober-minded and a little skinflint. They do not stand criticism, and they are quite good hosts in their families. Appropriate names are: Carmen, Kelly, Linda, Ariel, Henry, Sean, Ryan, Vincent.

November

November people are rather sagacious, being ready to improper deeds because of their personal benefit. They are mercenary and envious. These people are parsimonious, even for those who are closest to them. They do not like, however, being stingy with themselves. They may leave on holiday with their last money, although their families will have to starve long after that because of it. Women are narcissist, untidy and egotistical. They are leaders in their families and they do not consider their husbands' options into consideration, often being unfaithful to them even not trying to conceal this fact. They are sensuous and they do not choose their partners too much. They select weak-willed men, who have to endure too much from their wives. Men born in November often sink into depression and go through nervous crises. Appropriate names are: Jane, Chelsey, Megan, Pamela, Cody, Jared, Raymond, Gregory, Kenneth.

December

December people are distinguished for their enhanced emotionality, certain instability and quick temper over trifles. They are masters of themselves with difficulty when being irritated. Moreover, although they perfectly see shortcomings of theirs, and understand the motivations for the sometimes - negative attitude of the people surrounding them, they are not able to restrain themselves. Their lives are arranged in a complicated manner, they often find themselves in unpleasant situations. They cannot and do not know how to live their lives calmly. They sharply need frequent change of the atmosphere, the circle of communication and they do not endure monotonous way of living. They are subjected to emotional collapses and depressions. Appropriate names are: Gabriela, Lindsay, Abigail, Olivia, Elizabeth, Brian, Daniel,William.

Birthdays of Famous People

January

Famous People born on January 1st

1895 J. Edgar Hoover (founded FBI)
1909 Barry Goldwater (US senator and Republican Presidential Candidate)
1919 J.D. Salinger (author)

Famous People born on January 2nd

1967 {Tia Carrere (actress)

Famous People born on January 3rd

1892 J.R.R. Tolkien (author, Lord of the Rings, The Hobbit, etc)
1956 Mel Gibson (actor)

Famous People born on January 4th

1785 Jakob Grimm (author)
1960 Michael Stipe (singer)

Famous People born on January 5th

1931 Robert Duvall (actor)
1946 Diane Keaton (actress)
1969 Marilyn Manson (singer)

Famous People born on January 6th

1412 Joan of Arc (French national heroine, Roman Catholic saint)
1955 Rowan Atkinson (comedian, actor)

Famous People born on January 7th

1964 Nicolas Cage (actor)

Famous People born on January 8th

1937 Shirley Bassey (singer)
1947 David Bowie (singer)

Famous People born on January 9th

1913 Richard Nixon (37th US President)

1941 Joan Baez (singer)

Famous People born on January 10th

1945 Rod Stewart (singer)
1953 Pat Benatar (singer)

Famous People born on January 11th

1755 Alexander Hamilton (statesman)
1930 Rod Taylor (actor)

Famous People born on January 12th

1876 Jack London (author)
1951 Rush Limbaugh (radio presenter)
1954 Howard Stern (radio presenter)
1955 Kirstie Alley (actress)

Famous People born on January 13th

1919 Robert Stack (actor)

Famous People born on January 14th

1741 Benedict Arnold (traitorous General in the American Revolution)
1875 Albert Schweitzer (humanitarian, physician, musician, philospher)
1941 Faye Dunaway (actress)
1968 LL Cool J (rap singer)

Famous People born on January 15th

1870 Pierre S. DuPont (industrialist)
1908 Edward Teller (physicist, father of the "Hydrogen Bomb")
1913 Lloyd Bridges (actor)
1929 Dr. Martin Luther King, Jr. (civil rights leader)

Famous People born on January 16th

1909 Ethel Merman (actress, singer)
1948 John Carpenter (film director)
1974 Kate Moss (model)
1979 Aaliyah (singer, actress)

Famous People born on January 17th

1706 Benjamin Franklin (statesman, author, inventor)
1899 Al Capone (gangster)
1931 James Earl Jones (actor)
1942 Muhammad Ali, born Cassius Clay (boxer)

1962 Jim Carrey (comedian, actor)

Famous People born on January 18th

1779 Peter Roget (created the Thesaurus)
1882 A. A. Milne (author)
1892 Oliver Hardy (comedian, actor)
1904 Cary Grant (actor)
1955 Kevin Costner (actor)

Famous People born on January 19th

1736 James Watt (inventor)
1807 Robert E. Lee (Confederate General)
1809 Edgar Allan Poe (author, poet)
1943 Janis Joplin (singer)
1946 Dolly Parton (singer, actress)
1949 Robert Palmer (singer)

Famous People born on January 20th

1896 George Burns (comedian)
1930 Buzz Aldrin (astronaut)
1946 David Lynch (film director)

Famous People born on January 21st

1824 Stonewall Jackson (Confederate General)
1905 Christian Dior (fashion designer)
1924 Telly Savalas (actor)
1940 Jack Nicklaus (golfer)
1941 Placido Domingo (opera singer)
1950 Billy Ocean (singer)
1957 Geena Davis (actress)

Famous People born on January 22nd

1875 D.W. Griffith (film producer)
1935 Sam Cooke (singer)
1940 John Hurt (actor)

Famous People born on January 23rd

1944 Rutger Hauer (actor)
1957 Princess Caroline of Monaco

Famous People born on January 24th

1917 Ernest Borgnine (actor)
1941 Neil Diamond (singer)
1949 John Belushi (comedian, actor)

Famous People born on January 25th
1933 Corazon Aquino (President of Philippines)

Famous People born on January 26th
1880 Douglas MacArthur (US General)
1925 Paul Newman (actor)
1955 Eddie Van Halen (guitarist)
1958 Ellen DeGeneres (comedienne, actress)

Famous People born on January 27th
1756 Wolfgang Amadeus Mozart (composer)
1832 Lewis Caroll (author)
1964 Bridget Fonda (actress)

Famous People born on January 28th
1912 Jackson Pollock (artist)
1936 Alan Alda (actor)

Famous People born on January 29th
1880 W.C.Fields (comedian)
1843 William McKinley (25th US President)
1954 Oprah Winfrey (TV presenter)
1945 Tom Selleck (actor)

Famous People born on January 30th
1882 Franklin D. Roosevelt (32nd US President)
1930 Gene Hackman (actor)
1937 Vanessa Redgrave (actress)
1941 Richard B. Cheney (US Vice President)

Famous People born on January 31st
1919 Jackie Robinson (baseball player)
1923 Norman Mailer (author)

February

Famous People born on February 1st
1901 Clark Gable (actor)
1931 Boris Yeltsin (Russian President)
1965 Brandon Lee (actor)

Famous People born on February 2nd
1882 James Joyce (author)

1905 Ayn Rand (author)
1947 Farah Fawcett (actress)

Famous People born on February 3rd
1950 Morgan Fairchild (actress)

Famous People born on February 4th
1902 Charles Lindbergh (aviator)
1948 Alice Cooper (singer)
1975 Natalie Imbruglia (singer)

Famous People born on February 5th
1914 William Burroughs (author)
1948 Barbara Hershey (actress)
1962 Jennifer Jason Leigh (actress)

Famous People born on February 6th
1895 Babe Ruth (baseball player)
1911 Ronald W. Reagan (40th US President)
1945 Bob Marley (singer)

Famous People born on February 7th
1812 Charles Dickens (author)
1966 Chris Rock (comedian)

Famous People born on February 8th
1828 Jules Verne (author)
1925 Jack Lemmon (actor)
1931 James Dean (actor)

Famous People born on February 9th
1773 William Henry Harrison (9th US President)
1943 Joe Pesci (actor)
1945 Mia Farrow (actress)

Famous People born on February 10th
1893 Jimmy Durante (comedian, singer)
1930 Robert Wagner (actor)
1967 Laura Dern (actress)

Famous People born on February 11th

1847 Thomas Alva Edison (inventor)
1969 Jennifer Aniston (actress)

Famous People born on February 12th
1809 Abraham Lincoln (16th US President)
1809 Charles Darwin (scientist)

Famous People born on February 13th
1923 Chuck Yeager (aviator)
1944 Jerry Springer (TV presenter)
1950 Peter Gabriel (singer)
1974 Robbie Williams (singer)

Famous People born on February 14th
1894 Jack Benny (comedian)
1913 Jimmy Hoffa (labor leader)

Famous People born on February 15th
1564 Galileo Galilei (astronomer, scientist)
1951 Jane Seymour (actress)

Famous People born on February 16th
1958 Ice-T (rap singer, actor)
1959 John McEnroe (tennis player)

Famous People born on February 17th
1925 Hal Holbrook (actor)
1963 Michael Jordan (basketball player)

Famous People born on February 18th
1920 Jack Palance (actor)
1933 Yoko Ono (singer)
1954 John Travolta (actor)

Famous People born on February 19th
1473 Nicolas Copernicus (astronomer)
1924 Lee Marvin (actor)
1960 Prince Andrew, Duke of York (British royal)

Famous People born on February 20th
1924 Sidney Poitier (actor)

1954 Patty Hearst (kidnap victim)
1966 Cindy Crawford (model)
1967 Kurt Cobain (singer)

Famous People born on February 21st
1946 Tyne Daly (actress)
1955 Kelsey Grammer (actor)

Famous People born on February 22nd
1732 George Washinton (1st US President)
1975 Drew Barrymore (actress)

Famous People born on February 23rd
No names on this date

Famous People born on February 24th
1955 Steve Jobs (founded Apple Computer)
1966 Billy Zane (actor)

Famous People born on February 25th
1943 George Harrison (musician)

Famous People born on February 26th
1829 Levi Strauss (founded Levi Strauss!)
1932 Johnny Cash (singer)
1953 Michael Bolton (singer)

Famous People born on February 27th
1932 Elizabeth Taylor (actress)
1934 Ralph Nader (consumer advocate)

Famous People born on February 28th
1901 Linus Pauling (scientist)
1942 Brian Jones (musician)

Famous People born on February 29th
1860 Herman Hollerith (inventor - punched cards)

March

Famous People born on March 1st
1904 Glenn Miller (musician)

1910 David Niven (actor)
1927 Harry Belafonte (singer)
1944 Roger Daltrey (singer, actor)

Famous People born on March 2nd

1904 Theodor Seuss Giesel, "Dr Seuss" (author)
1931 Mikhail Gorbachev (Soviet leader)
1944 Lou Reed (singer)
1962 Jon Bon Jovi (singer)

Famous People born on March 3rd

1847 Alexander Graham Bell (inventor)
1920 James Doohan (actor)

Famous People born on March 4th

1678 Antonio Vivaldi (composer)
1962 Patsy Kensit (actress, singer)

Famous People born on March 5th

1908 Rex Harrison (actor)
1936 Dean Stockwell (actor)
1958 Andy Gibb (singer)

Famous People born on March 6th

1475 Michelangelo (artist)
1926 Alan Greenspan (economist, chairman of Federal Reserve)
1944 Kiri Te Kanawa (opera singer)

Famous People born on March 7th

1930 Lord Snowdon (photographer)
1960 Ivan Lendl (tennis player)

Famous People born on March 8th

1943 Lynn Redgrave (actress)
1963 Kathy Ireland (actress)
1976 Freddie Prinze, Jr. (musician)

Famous People born on March 9th

1918 Mickey Spillane (author)
1934 Yuri Gagarin (astronaut)
1940 Raul Julia (actor)
1943 Bobby Fischer (chess player)

Famous People born on March 10th

1940 Chuck Norris (actor)
1958 Sharon Stone (actress)
1964 Prince Edward, Earl of Wessex (British royal)

Famous People born on March 11th

1931 Rupert Murdoch (media mogul)
1950 Bobby McFerrin (singer)
1952 Douglas Adams (author)

Famous People born on March 12th

1946 Liza Minnelli (actress, singer)
1948 James Taylor (musician)

Famous People born on March 13th

1733 Joseph Priestly (scientist: first to isolate oxygen)
1855 Percival Lowell (astronomer)
1911 L. Ron Hubbard (author, founder of Church of Scientology)
1939 Neil Sedaka (singer)

Famous People born on March 14th

1879 Albert Einstein (scientist)
1933 Michael Caine (actor)
1947 Billy Crystal (actor)

Famous People born on March 15th

1767 Andrew Jackson (7th US President)
1933 Quincy Jones (musician, record producer)
1944 Sly Stone (musician)

Famous People born on March 16th

1751 James Madison (4th US President)
1926 Jerry Lewis (actor, comedian)
1949 Erik Estrada (actor)

Famous People born on March 17th

1919 Nat "King Cole" (singer)
1938 Rudolf Nureyev (ballet dancer)
1949 Patrick Duffy (actor)
1951 Kurt Russell (actor)
1964 Rob Lowe (actor)

Famous People born on March 18th
1837 Grover Cleveland (22nd and 24th US President)
1936 Fredrik Willem de Klerk (South African President)
1941 Wilson Pickett (singer)
1963 Vanessa Williams (singer, actress)
1970 Queen Latifah (singer)

Famous People born on March 19th
1928 Patrick McGoohan (actor)
1936 Ursula Andress (actress)
1947 Glenn Close (actress)
1955 Bruce Willis (actor)

Famous People born on March 20th
1957 Spike Lee (film director)
1958 Holly Hunter(actress)

Famous People born on March 21st
1944 Timothy Dalton (actor)
1958 Gary Oldman (actor)
1962 Matthew Broderick (actor)

Famous People born on March 22nd
1887 Chico Marx (comedian)
1931 William Shatner (actor)
1948 Andrew Lloyd Weber (composer)
1976 Reese Witherspoon (actress)

Famous People born on March 23rd
1910 Akira Kurosawa (film director)
1912 Wernher Von Braun (rocket scientist)
1929 Roger Bannister (runner)
1953 Chaka Khan (singer)

Famous People born on March 24th
1874 Harry Houdini (escapologist)
1930 Steve McQueen (actor)

Famous People born on March 25th
1942 Aretha Franklin (singer)
1947 Elton John (singer)
1965 Sarah Jessica Parker (actress)

Famous People born on March 26th

Tennessee Williams (writer)
1931 Leonard Nimoy (actor)
1939 James Caan (actor)
1944 Diana Ross (singer)
1950 Martin Short (actor)

Famous People born on March 27th

1942 Michael York (actor)
1963 Quentin Tarantino (film director)
1970 Mariah Carey (singer)

Famous People born on March 28th

1921 Dirk Bogarde (actor)

Famous People born on March 29th

1790 John Tyler (10th US President)
1943 John Major (former British Prime Minister)
1964 Elle Macpherson (model)
1968 Lucy Lawless (actress)

Famous People born on March 30th

1746 Francisco Goya (artist)
1853 Vincent Van Gogh (artist)
1937 Warren Beatty (actor)
1945 Eric Clapton (musician)
1962 M.C. Hammer (singer)
1968 Celine Dion (singer)

Famous People born on March 31st

1596 Rene Descartes (philospher)
1732 Joseph Haydn (composer)
1948 Al Gore (US Vice President)
1971 Ewan McGregor (actor)

April

Famous People born on April 1st

1938 Ali MacGraw (actress)

Famous People born on April 2nd

1805 Hans Christian Andersen (author)
1914 Sir Alec Guinness (actor)
1939 Marvin Gaye (singer)

Famous People born on April 3rd
1942 Wayne Newton (singer)
1958 Alec Baldwin (actor)
1961 Eddie Murphy (comedian, actor)

Famous People born on April 4th
1915 Muddy Waters (musician)
1932 Anthony Perkins (actor)

Famous People born on April 5th
1900 Spencer Tracy (actor)
1908 Bette Davis (actress)
1916 Gregory Peck (actor)

Famous People born on April 6th
1929 Andre Previn (pianist, composer)
1952 Marilu Henner (actress)

Famous People born on April 7th
1915 Billie Holiday (singer)
1928 James Garner (actor)
1939 Francis Ford Coppola (film director)
1954 Jackie Chan (actor)

Famous People born on April 8th
1938 Kofi Annan (UN Secretary General)
1963 Julian Lennon (singer)
1968 Patricia Arquette (actress)

Famous People born on April 9th
1926 Hugh Hefner (founder of Playboy)

Famous People born on April 10th
1794 Commodore Matthew Perry (explorer)
1929 Max Von Sydow (actor)
1932 Omar Sherif (actor)
1952 Steven Seagal (actor)

Famous People born on April 11th
1966 Lisa Stansfield (singer)

Famous People born on April 12th

1940 Herbie Hancock (musician)
1947 Tom Clancy (author)
1956 Andy Garcia (actor)
1971 Shannen Doherty (actress)

Famous People born on April 13th

1743 Thomas Jefferson (3rd US President)
1963 Garry Kasparov (chess player)

Famous People born on April 14th

1904 John Gielgud (actor)
1941 Julie Christie (actress)
1945 Ritchie Blackmore (guitarist)
1977 Sarah Michelle Gellar (actress)

Famous People born on April 15th

1452 Leonardo da Vinci (artist, visionary)
1966 Samantha Fox (singer, model)

Famous People born on April 16th

1921 Peter Ustinov (actor)
1939 Dusty Springfield (singer)

Famous People born on April 17th

1894 Nikita Krushchev (Soviet leader)
1974 Victoria Beckham, "Posh Spice" (singer)

Famous People born on April 18th

1947 James Woods (actor)
1963 Conan O'Brien (TV presenter)

Famous People born on April 19th

1935 Dudley Moore (actor, comedian)
1946 Tim Curry (actor)

Famous People born on April 20th

1889 Adolf Hitler (German dictator)
1893 Harold Lloyd (actor)
1949 Jessica Lange (actress)
1972 Carmen Electra (singer, model, actress)

Famous People born on April 21st
1816 Charlotte Bronte (author)
1926 Queen Elizabeth II (British Queen)
1947 Iggy Pop (singer)
1958 Andie Macdowell (actress)

Famous People born on April 22nd
1870 Vladimir Ilyich Lenin (revolutionary, Soviet leader)
1928 Aaron Spelling (TV producer)
1937 Jack Nicholson (actor)

Famous People born on April 23rd
1564 William Shakespeare (playwright)
1791 James Buchanan (15th US President)
1936 Roy Orbison (singer)
1940 Lee Majors (actor)

Famous People born on April 24th
1934 Shirley MacLaine (actress)
1936 Jill Ireland (actress)
1942 Barbra Streisand (singer, actress)

Famous People born on April 25th
1918 Ella Fitzgerald (singer)
1940 Al Pacino (actor)

Famous People born on April 26th
1938 Duane Eddy (guitarist)

Famous People born on April 27th
1822 Ulysses S. Grant (18th US President)
1959 Sheena Easton (singer)

Famous People born on April 28th
1758 James Monroe (5th US President)
1937 Saddam Hussein (Iraqi President)
1950 Jay Leno (TV presenter)

Famous People born on April 29th
1769 Arthur Wellesley, Duke of Wellington (British General, battle of Waterloo, later British Prime Minister)
1970 Uma Thurman (actress)

1970 Andre Agassi (tennis player)

Famous People born on April 30th

1933 Willie Nelson (singer, actor)

May

Famous People born on May 1st

1945 Rita Coolidge (singer)

1967 Tim McGraw (singer)

Famous People born on May 2nd

1936 Engelbert Humperdinck (singer)

Famous People born on May 3rd

1898 Golda Meir (Israeli Prime Minister)

1933 James Brown (singer)

Famous People born on May 4th

1929 Audrey Hepburn (actress)

Famous People born on May 5th

1818 Karl Marx (author)

1942 Tammy Wynette (singer)

Famous People born on May 6th

1856 Sigmund Freud (founder of psychoanalysis)

1868 Tsar Nicholas II (last Russian Tsar, overthrown in Russian Revolution)

1953 Tony Blair (British Prime Minster)

1961 George Clooney (actor)

Famous People born on May 7th

1833 Johannes Brahms (composer)

1840 Peter Ilyich Tchaikovsky (composer)

1919 Eva Peron (wife of Argentine leader, Juan Peron)

Famous People born on May 8th

1884 Harry S. Truman (33rd US President)

1953 Alex Van Halen (musician)

Famous People born on May 9th

1936 Glenda Jackson (actress)

1949 Billy Joel (singer)

Famous People born on May 10th

1899 Fred Astaire (dancer, actor)
1960 Bono (singer)

Famous People born on May 11th
1904 Salvador Dali (artist)
1912 Phil Silvers (comedian)

Famous People born on May 12th
1820 Florence Nightingale (nurse)
1929 Burt Bacharach (singer)
1962 Emilio Estevez (actor)

Famous People born on May 13th
1914 Joe Louis (boxer)
1939 Harvey Keitel (actor)
1950 Stevie Wonder (singer, musician)

Famous People born on May 14th
1727 Thomas Gainsborough (artist)
1969 Cate Blanchett (actress)

Famous People born on May 15th
1930 Jasper Johns (artist)

Famous People born on May 16th
1966 Janet Jackson (singer)

Famous People born on May 17th
1902 Ayatollah Khomeini (Iranian leader)
1961 Enya (singer)

Famous People born on May 18th
1897 Frank Capra (film director)
1912 Perry Como (singer)

Famous People born on May 19th
1890 Ho Chi Minh (Vietnamese leader)
1925 Malcolm X (civil rights leader)
1945 Pete Townsend (musician)
1952 Grace Jones (model, singer, actress)

Famous People born on May 20th

1908 Jimmy Stewart (actor)
1944 Joe Cocker (singer)
1946 Cher (singer, actress)

Famous People born on May 21st

1688 Alexander Pope (poet)
1844 Henri Rosseau (artist)
1917 Raymond Burr (actor)
1952 Mr T. (actor)

Famous People born on May 22nd

1907 Sir Laurence Olivier (actor)

Famous People born on May 23rd

1707 Carl Linnaeus (scientist, "Father of Taxonomy")
1974 Jewel (singer)

Famous People born on May 24th

1819 Queen Victoria (British Queen 1837-1901)
1941 Bob Dylan (singer, poet)
1944 Patti LaBelle (singer)
1955 Rosanne Cash (singer)

Famous People born on May 25th

1927 Robert Ludlum (author)
1963 Mike Myers (actor, comedian)

Famous People born on May 26th

1907 John Wayne (actor)
1913 Peter Cushing (actor)
1948 Stevie Nicks (singer)
1949 Pam Grier (actress)
1964 Lenny Kravitz (singer)

Famous People born on May 27th

1911 Vincent Price (actor)
1923 Dr Henry Kissinger (US Secretary of State)
1936 Louis Gossett, Jr. (actor)
1971 Paul Bettany (actor)

Famous People born on May 28th

1807 Louis Agassiz (scientist, postulated "Ice Ages")
1908 Ian Fleming (author)
1968 Kylie Minogue (singer, actress)

Famous People born on May 29th
1903 Bob Hope (comedian)
1917 John F. Kennedy (35th US President)
1958 Annette Bening (actress)

Famous People born on May 30th
1908 Mel Blanc (cartoon voices)

Famous People born on May 31st
1922 Denholm Elliott (actor)
1930 Clint Eastwood (actor)
1943 Sharon Gless (actress)
1965 Brooke Shields (actress)

June

Famous People born on June 1st
1930 Edward Woodward (actor)
1974 Alanis Morissette (singer)

Famous People born on June 2nd
1941 Stacy Keach (actor)

Famous People born on June 3rd
1906 Josephine Baker (dancer)
1925 Tony Curtis (actor)
1950 Suzy Quatro (singer)

Famous People born on June 4th
1928 Dr Ruth Westheimer (therapist, author)
Famous People born on June 5th
1956 Kenny G (singer)

Famous People born on June 6th
1956 Bjorn Borg (tennis player)

Famous People born on June 7th
1917 Dean Martin (singer, actor)
1958 Prince (singer)
1981 Anna Kournikova (tennis player)

Famous People born on June 8th
1867 Frank Lloyd Wright (architect)

1925 Barbara P. Bush (former US first lady)

Famous People born on May 9th
1936 Glenda Jackson (actress)
1949 Billy Joel (singer)

Famous People born on June 10th
1921 Prince Philip, Duke of Edinburgh (British royal)
1966 Elizabeth Hurley (model, actress)

Famous People born on June 11th
1776 John Constable (artist)
1910 Jacques Costeau (diver)
1935 Gene Wilder (actor)

Famous People born on June 12th
1924 George Herbert Walker Bush (41st US President)
1929 Anne Frank (diarist)

Famous People born on June 13th
1865 William Butler Yeats (poet)

Famous People born on June 14th
1946 Donald Trump (business man)
1961 Boy George (singer)
1969 Steffi Graf (tennis player)

Famous People born on June 15th
1954 Jim Belushi (actor)
1963 Helen Hunt (actress)
1964 Courtney Cox (actress)

Famous People born on June 16th
1890 Stan Laurel (comedian, actor)
1971 Tupac Shakur (rap singer)

Famous People born on June 17th
1882 Igor Stravinsky (composer)
1946 Barry Manilow (singer)
1980 Venus Williams (tennis player)

Famous People born on June 18th
1942 Paul McCartney (singer)
1952 Isabella Rossellini (actress)

Famous People born on June 19th

1623 Blaise Pascal (mathematician)
1954 Kathleen Turner (actress)
1962 Paula Abdul (singer)

Famous People born on June 20th

1909 Errol Flynn (actor)
1931 Martin Landau (actor)
1949 Lionel Richie (singer)
1952 John Goodman (actor)

Famous People born on June 21st

1905 Jean-Paul Satre (philospher)
1921 Jane Russell (actress)
1982 Prince William (British royal)

Famous People born on June 22nd

1936 Kris Kristofferson (actor)
1949 Meryl Streep (actress)
1973 Carson Daly (MTV)

Famous People born on June 23rd

1929 June Carter (singer)

Famous People born on June 24th

1944 Jeff Beck (guitarist)

Famous People born on June 25th

1903 George Orwell (author)
1945 Carly Simon (singer)
1963 George Michael (singer)

Famous People born on June 26th

1970 Chris O'Donnell (actor)

Famous People born on June 27th

1880 Helen Keller (author, educator)

Famous People born on June 28th

1491 Henry VIII (King of England)
1902 John Dillinger (gangster)

1926 Mel Brooks (comedian, film director, actor)

Famous People born on June 29th

1901 Nelson Eddy (actor, singer)
1962 Amanda Donohoe (actress)

Famous People born on June 30th

1966 Mike Tyson (boxer)

July

Famous People born on July 1st

1916 Olivia DeHavilland (actress)
1945 Deborah Harry (singer, actress)
1952 Dan Aykroyd (comedian, actor)
1961 Carl Lewis (runner)
1967 Pamela Anderson (model, actress)

Famous People born on July 2nd

1908 Thurgood Marshall (first black US Supreme Court Justice)

Famous People born on July 3rd

1883 Franz Kafka (author)
1927 Ken Russell (film director)
1962 Tom Cruise (actor)

Famous People born on July 4th

1872 Calvin Coolidge (30th US President)
1938 Bill Withers (singer)
1962 Pam Shriver (tennis player)

Famous People born on July 5th

1810 P.T. Barnum (showman)
1911 Georges Pompidou (French President)

Famous People born on July 6th

1925 Bill Haley (singer)
1935 Dalai Lama (Tibetan leader)
1946 Sylvester Stallone (actor)
1946 George W. Bush (43rd US President)

Famous People born on July 7th

1940 Ringo Starr (musician)

Famous People born on July 8th

1951 Anjelica Huston (actress)
1958 Kevin Bacon (actor)

Famous People born on July 9th

1947 O.J.Simpson (American football player, actor)
1956 Tom Hanks (actor)
1957 Kelly McGillis (actress)
1964 Courtney Love (singer, actress)
1976 Fred Savage (actor)

Famous People born on July 10th

1945 Virginia Wade (tennis player)

Famous People born on July 11th

1767 John Quincy Adams (6th US President)
1959 Suzanne Vega (singer)

Famous People born on July 12th

1861 George Washington Carver (scientist)
1937 Bill Cosby (comedian, actor)

Famous People born on July 13th

100 BC Julius Caesar (Roman general leader)
1940 Patrick Stewart (actor)
1944 Erno Rubik (inventor of puzzles)

Famous People born on July 14th

1912 Woody Guthrie (singer)
1913 Gerald Ford (38th US President)

Famous People born on July 15th

1606 Rembrandt (artist)
1944 Jan-Michel Vincent (actor)
1946 Linda Ronstadt (singer)
1951 Jesse Ventura (wrestler, actor, politician)

Famous People born on July 16th

1872 Roald Amundsen (explorer)
1907 Barbara Stanwyck (actress)
1911 Ginger Rodgers (actress)

Famous People born on July 17th

1934 Donald Sutherland (actor)
1952 David Hasselhoff (actor, singer)

Famous People born on July 18th
1918 Nelson Mandela (South African President)
1938 Paul Verhoeven (film director)
Famous People born on July 19th
1947 Brian May (guitarist)

Famous People born on July 20th
1804 Sir Richard Owen (scientist, coined the term "Dinosaur")
1919 Sir Edmund Hillary (mountaineer)
1938 Diana Rigg (actress)
1947 Carlos Santana (guitarist)

Famous People born on July 21st
1899 Ernest Hemingway (author)
1948 Cat Stevens (singer)
1952 Robin Williams (actor, comedian)

Famous People born on July 22nd
1947 Danny Glover (actor)

Famous People born on July 23rd
1961 Woody Harrelson (actor)
1973 Monica Lewinsky (Whitehouse intern)

Famous People born on July 24th
1783 Simon Bolivar (revolutionary)
1951 Lynda Carter (actress)
1970 Jennifer Lopez (singer, actress)

Famous People born on July 25th
1967 Matt LeBlanc (actor)

Famous People born on July 26th
1875 Carl Jung (psychiatrist)
1894 Aldous Huxley (author)
1943 Mick Jagger (singer, actor)
1959 Kevin Spacey (actor)

Famous People born on July 27th
1916 Kennan Wynn (actor)
1937 Don Galloway (actor)

1944 Bobbie Gentry (singer)

Famous People born on July 28th

1866 Beatrix Potter (author)

Famous People born on July 29th

1871 Grigori Rasputin (Russian priest)
1883 Benito Mussolini (Italian dictator)

Famous People born on July 30th

1818 Emily Bronte (author)
1863 Henry Ford (founder of Ford Motor Company)
1947 Arnold Schwarzenegger (actor)
1963 Lisa Kudrow (actress)

Famous People born on July 31st

1912 Milton Friedman (economist)
1951 Evonne Goolagong Cawley (tennis player)
1962 Wesley Snipes (actor)
1966 Dean Cain (actor)

August

Famous People born on August 1st

1744 Jean-Baptiste Lamarck (scientist)
1942 Jerry Garcia (musician)
1963 Coolio (singer)

Famous People born on August 2nd

1932 Peter O'Toole (actor)

Famous People born on August 3rd

1926 Tony Bennett (singer)
1940 Martin Sheen (actor)

Famous People born on August 4th

1901 Louis Armstrong (musician, singer)

Famous People born on August 5th

1930 Neil Armstrong (astronaut)

Famous People born on August 6th

1809 Alfred Lord Tennyson (poet)
1911 Lucille Ball (actress, comedienne)
1917 Robert Mitchum (actor)
1928 Andy Warhol (artist, film director)
1972 Geri Halliwell, "Ginger Spice" (singer)

Famous People born on August 7th
1876 Mata Hari (spy)
1960 David Duchovny (actor)

Famous People born on August 8th
1937 Dustin Hoffman (actor)

Famous People born on August 9th
1896 Jean Piaget (psychologist)
1957 Melanie Griffith (actress)
1963 Whitney Houston (singer, actress)

Famous People born on August 10th
1874 Herbert Hoover (31st US President)
1959 Rosanna Arquette (actress)

Famous People born on August 11th
1933 Reverend Jerry Falwell (evangalist)
1950 Steve Wozniak (founder Apple Computer)

Famous People born on August 12th
1881 Cecil B. DeMille (film director)
1949 Mark Knopfler (guitarist, singer)
1971 Pete Sampras (tennis player)

Famous People born on August 13th
1899 Alfred Hitchcock (film director)
1926 Fidel Castro (Cuban leader)

Famous People born on August 14th
1968 Halle Berry (actress)

Famous People born on August 15th
1769 Napoleon Bonaparte (French Emperor)
1950 Princess Anne, The Princess Royal (British royal)
1972 Ben Affleck (actor)

Famous People born on August 16th
1913 Menachem Begin (Israeli Prime Minister)
1954 James Cameron (film director)
1958 Madonna (singer, actress)

Famous People born on August 17th
1943 Robert De Niro (actor)
1960 Sean Penn (actor)

Famous People born on August 18th
1933 Roman Polanski (film director)
1937 Robert Redford (actor)
1954 Patrick Swayze (actor)

Famous People born on August 19th
1871 Orville Wright (aviator)
1883 Coco Chanel (fashion designer, perfume creator)
1921 Gene Roddenberry (creator of Startrek)
1946 William J. Clinton (42nd US President)

Famous People born on August 20th
1833 Benjamin Harrison (23rd US President)
1890 H.P. Lovecraft (author)
1948 Robert Plant (singer)

Famous People born on August 21st
1938 Kenny Rodgers (singer, actor)
1956 Kim Cattrall (actress)

Famous People born on August 22nd
1862 Claude Debussy (composer)
1904 Deng Xiaoping (Chinese leader)
1920 Ray Bradbury (author)

Famous People born on August 23rd
1769 Georges Cuvier (scientist, established the fact of extinction)
1912 Gene Kelly (actor)
1949 Shelley Long (actress)
1970 River Phoenix (actor)

Famous People born on August 24th
1929 Yasser Arafat (Palestinian leader)
1958 Steve Guttenberg (actor)

Famous People born on August 25th

1930 Sean Connery (actor)
1954 Elvis Costello (singer)
1970 Claudia Schiffer (model)

Famous People born on August 26th

1743 Antoine Lavoisier (scientist)
1980 Macaulay Culkin (actor)

Famous People born on August 27th

1908 Lyndon B. Johnson (36th US President)
1910 Mother Teresa (humanitarian)
1947 Barbara Bach (actress)
1952 Paul Reubens, "Peewee Herman" (actor)

Famous People born on August 28th

1943 David Soul (actor, singer)
1965 Shania Twain (singer)

Famous People born on August 29th

1915 Ingrid Bergman (actress)
1938 Elliot Gould (actor)
1958 Michael Jackson (singer)

Famous People born on August 30th

1972 Cameron Diaz (model, actress)

Famous People born on August 31st

1945 Van Morrison (singer)
1970 Debbie Gibson (singer)

September

Famous People born on September 1st

1875 Edgar Rice Burroughs (author)
1939 Lily Tomlin (actress)
1957 Gloria Estefan (singer)

Famous People born on September 2nd

1952 Jimmy Connors (tennis player)
1964 Keanu Reeves (actor)
1968 Salma Hayek (actress)

Famous People born on September 3rd
1965 Charlie Sheen (actor)

Famous People born on September 4th
1917 Henry Ford II (businessman)
1970 Ione Skye (actress)

Famous People born on September 5th
1940 Raquel Welch (actress)
1946 Freddie Mercury (singer)

Famous People born on September 6th
1973 Greg Rusedski (tennis player)

Famous People born on September 7th
1936 Buddy Holly (singer)
1949 Gloria Gaynor (singer)
1951 Chrissie Hynde (singer)
1954 Corbin Bernsen (actor)

Famous People born on September 8th
1925 Peter Sellers (actor, comedian)
1979 Pink (singer)

Famous People born on September 9th
1941 Otis Redding (singer)
1951 Michael Keaton (actor)
1960 Hugh Grant (actor)

Famous People born on September 10th
1953 Amy Irving (actress)

Famous People born on September 11th
1967 Harry Connick, Jr. (actor, singer)

Famous People born on September 12th
1888 Maurice Chevalier (singer)
1913 Jesse Owens (athlete)

Famous People born on September 13th
1860 John J. Pershing (US General)
1925 Mel Torme (singer)

Famous People born on September 14th

1849 Ivan Pavlov (scientist)

Famous People born on September 15th

1857 Howard Taft (27th US President)
1946 Oliver Stone (film director)
1946 Tommy Lee Jones (actor)
1984 Prince Henry "Harry" (British royal)

Famous People born on September 16th

1925 B.B. King (singer)
1956 Mickey Rourke (actor)
1956 David Copperfield (magician)

Famous People born on September 17th

1928 Roddy McDowall (actor)
1931 Anne Bancroft (actress)

Famous People born on September 18th

1905 Greta Garbo (actress)
1939 Frankie Avalon (singer)

Famous People born on September 19th

1933 David McCallum (actor)
1948 Jeremy Irons (actor)
1949 Leslie Lawson, "Twiggy" (model, actress)

Famous People born on September 20th

1934 Sophia Loren (actress)

Famous People born on September 21st

1866 H.G. Wells (author, visionary)
1931 Larry Hagman (actor)
1947 Stephen King (author)
1968 Ricki Lake (TV presenter, actress)

Famous People born on September 22nd

1957 Nick Cave (singer)

Famous People born on September 23rd

63 BC Augustus Caesar (first Roman emperor)
1943 Julio Iglesias (singer)
1949 Bruce Springsteen (singer)

Famous People born on September 24th

1936 Jim Henson (creator the "The Muppets")
1941 Linda McCartney (photographer, singer)

Famous People born on September 25th

1944 Michael Douglas (actor)
1951 Mark Hamill (actor)
1952 Christopher Reeve (actor)
1961 Heather Locklear (actress)
1968 Will Smith (actor, singer)
1969 Catherine Zeta-Jones (actress)

Famous People born on September 26th

1888 T.S Eliot (author)
1898 George Gershwin (composer)
1948 Olivia Newton-John (singer, actress)
1962 Lawrence Leritz (Actor, Producer, Dancer. Time Magazine honored Leritz as their Local Hero 1996 for his work) - information provided by his brother, Len Leritz.
1981 Serena Williams (tennis player)

Famous People born on September 27th

1958 Shaun Cassidy (actor, singer)

Famous People born on September 28th

1573 Caravaggio (artist)
1934 Brigitte Bardot (actress)
1967 Mira Sorvino (actress)
1972 Gwyneth Paltrow (actress)

Famous People born on September 29th

1931 Anita Ekberg (actress)
1935 Jerry Lee Lewis (singer)
1942 Ian Mcshane (actor)
1943 Lech Walesa (Polish labor leader, later President)
1960 Jennifer Rush (singer)

Famous People born on September 30th

1931 Angie Dickinson (actress)
1935 Johnny Mathis (singer)

October

Famous People born on October 1st

1920 Walter Matthau (actor)
1924 Jimmy Carter (39th US President)
1928 George Peppard (actor)
1935 Julie Andrews (actress, singer)

Famous People born on October 2nd
1869 Mahatma Gandhi (Indian leader)
1951 Sting (singer)

Famous People born on October 3rd
1925 Gore Vidal (author)
1941 Chubby Checker (singer)
1962 Tommy Lee (drummer in Motley Crue, Pamela Anderson's ex)
1973 Neve Campbell (actress)

Famous People born on October 4th
1822 Rutherford B. Hayes (19th US President)
1924 Charlton Heston (actor)
1946 Susan Sarandon (actress)
1976 Alicia Silverstone (actress)

Famous People born on October 5th
1902 Ray Kroc (founder McDonalds)
1902 Larry Fine (of The Three Stooges)
1919 Donald Pleasence (actor)
1954 Sir Bob Geldof (singer, actor, TV presenter, humanitarian)
1975 Kate Winslet (actress)

Famous People born on October 6th
1942 Britt Ekland (actress)

Famous People born on October 7th
1885 Niels Bohr (scientist)
Bishop Desmond Tutu (anti-apartheid campaigner)
1952 Vladimir Putin (Russian President)

Famous People born on October 8th
1895 Juan Peron (Argentine President)
1941 Jesse Jackson (civil rights leader, US Presidential Candidate)
1943 Chevy Chase (comedian)
1949 Sigourney Weaver (actress)

Famous People born on October 9th
1940 John Lennon (singer, musician)

Famous People born on October 10th
1813 Giuseppe Verdi (composer)
1930 Harold Pinter (playwright)
1955 David Lee Roth (singer)

Famous People born on October 11th
1966 Luke Perry (actor)

Famous People born on October 12th
1935 Luciano Pavarotti (opera singer)

Famous People born on October 13th
1925 Margaret Thatcher (former British Prime Minster)
1947 Sammy Hagar (singer)
1959 Marie Osmond (singer)

Famous People born on October 14th
1890 Dwight D. Eisenhower (US general, 34th US President)
1927 Roger Moore (actor)
1939 Ralph Lauren (fashion designer)
1940 Cliff Richard (singer)

Famous People born on October 15th
1917 Arthur Schlesinger, Jr. (historian)
1924 Lee Iacocca (businessman)

Famous People born on October 16th
1854 Oscar Wilde (author)
1925 Angela Lansbury (actress)

Famous People born on October 17th
1938 Evel Knievel (motorcycle stuntman)

Famous People born on October 18th
1926 Chuck Berry (singer, guitarist)
1956 Martina Navratilova (tennis player)
1960 Jean-Claude Van Damme (actor)

Famous People born on October 19th
1931 John Le Carre (author)
1945 John Lithgow (actor)

Famous People born on October 20th
1953 Tom Petty (singer)

1972 Snoop Doggy Dogg (rap singer)

Famous People born on October 21st

1949 Benjamin Netanyahu (Israeli Prime Minister)
1956 Carrie Fisher (actress)

Famous People born on October 22nd

1811 Franz Liszt (composer)
1938 Christopher Lloyd (actor)
1943 Catherine Deneuve (actress)
1952 Jeff Goldblum (actor)

Famous People born on October 23rd

1940 Pele (soccer player)
1942 Michael Crichton (author)
1959 "Weird" Al Yankovic (comedian, actor, singer)

Famous People born on October 24th

1947 Kevin Kline (actor)

Famous People born on October 25th

1838 Georges Bizet (composer)
1881 Pablo Picasso (artist)

Famous People born on October 26th

1942 Bob Hoskins (actor)
1947 Hillary Rodham Clinton (former US first lady, US senator)

Famous People born on October 27th

1858 Theodore Roosevelt (naturalist, explorer, adventurer, big game hunter, 1906 Nobel Peace Prize Winner and 26th US President!)
1914 Dylan Thomas (books)
1923 Roy Lichtenstein (artist)
1939 John Cleese (actor, comedian)

Famous People born on October 28th

1955 Bill Gates (founder Microsoft)
1967 Julia Roberts (actress)

Famous People born on October 29th

1947 Richard Dreyfuss (actor)
1971 Winona Ryder (actress)

Famous People born on October 30th

1735 John Adams (2nd US President)
1939 Grace Slick (singer)
1951 Harry Hamlin (actor)
1960 Diego Armando Maradona (soccer player)

Famous People born on October 31st
1795 John Keats (poet)
1887 Chiang Kai-Shek (Chinese leader)
1931 Dan Rather (news broadcaster, journalist)
1950 John Candy (actor, comedian)

November

Famous People born on November 1st
1972 Jenny McCarthy (TV presenter, model, actress)

Famous People born on November 2nd
1795 James K. Polk (11th US President)
1865 Warren Harding (29th US President)
1913 Burt Lancaster (actor)
1942 Stefanie Powers (actress)

Famous People born on November 3rd
1921 Charles Bronson (actor)
1954 Adam Ant (singer)
1959 Dolph Lundgren (actor)

Famous People born on November 4th
1937 Loretta Swift (actress)
1946 Laura Welch Bush (US 1st lady)

Famous People born on November 5th
1940 Elke Sommer (actress)
1963 Tatum O'Neal (actress)

Famous People born on November 6th
1946 Sally Field (actress)
1970 Ethan Hawke (actor)

Famous People born on November 7th
1867 Marie Curie (scientist)

Famous People born on November 8th
1847 Bram Stoker (author)

1949 Bonnie Raitt (singer)

Famous People born on November 9th

1934 Carl Sagan (scientist, author)

Famous People born on November 10th

1483 Martin Luther (founded Protestant movement)
1925 Richard Burton (actor)
1935 Roy Scheider (actor)

Famous People born on November 11th

1962 Demi Moore (actress)
1974 Leonardo DiCaprio (actor)

Famous People born on November 12th

1945 Neil Young (singer)
1966 David Schwimmer (actor)

Famous People born on November 13th

354 Saint Augustine (writer, theologian, Catholic Saint)
1850 Robert Louis Stevenson (author)

Famous People born on November 14th

1840 Claude Monet (artist)
1889 Jawaharlal Nehru (Indian Prime Minister)
1922 Boutros Boutros-Ghali (UN Secretary General)
1948 Charles, Prince of Wales (British royal)

Famous People born on November 15th

1929 Ed Asner (actor)
1932 Petula Clark (singer)

Famous People born on November 16th

1967 Lisa Bonet (actress)

Famous People born on November 17th

1925 Rock Hudson (actor)
1942 Martin Scorsese (film director)
1944 Danny DeVito (actor)

Famous People born on November 18th

1836 Sir William Gilbert (composer)
1901 George Gallup (pollster)
1923 Alan Shepard, Jr. (astronaut)

1942 Linda Evans (actress)

Famous People born on November 19th

1831 James Garfield (20th US President)
1917 Indira Gandhi (Indian Prime Minister)
1942 Calvin Klein (fashion designer)
1961 Meg Ryan (actress)
1962 Jodie Foster (actress)

Famous People born on November 20th

1956 Bo Derek (actress)

Famous People born on November 21st

1898 Rene Magritte (artist)
1965 Bjork (singer)

Famous People born on November 22nd

1890 Charles de Gaulle (French General, wartime leader, later President)
1913 Benjamin Britten (composer)
1932 Robert Vaughn (actor)
1943 Billie Jean King (tennis player)
1958 Jamie Lee Curtis (actress)

Famous People born on November 23rd

1804 Franklin Pierce (14th US President)
1859 Billy the Kid (gunslinger)
1887 Boris Karloff (actor)
1888 Harpo Marx (comedian)

Famous People born on November 24th

1784 Zachary Taylor (12th US President)
1864 Toulouse-Lautrec (artist)
1868 Scott Joplin (musician)
1925 William F. Buckley Jr. (founder of National Review)

Famous People born on November 25th

1914 Joe DiMaggio (baseball player)
1920 Ricardo Montalban (actor)
1971 Christina Applegate (actress)

Famous People born on November 26th

1922 Charles Schulz (cartoonist)
1939 Tina Turner (singer)

Famous People born on November 27th
1940 Bruce Lee (actor)
1942 Jimi Hendrix (singer, guitarist)
1964 Robin Givens (model, actress)

Famous People born on November 28th
1757 William Blake (poet, artist)
1950 Ed Harris (actor)
1967 Anna Nicole Smith (model, actress)

Famous People born on November 29th
1898 C. S. Lewis (author)
1949 Gary Shandling (comedian, actor)
1956 Jeff Fahey (actor)

Famous People born on November 30th
1667 Jonathan Swift (author, satirist)
1835 Mark Twain (author)
1874 Sir Winston Churchill (British Prime Minister)
1955 Billy Idol (singer)

December

Famous People born on December 1st
1935 Woody Allen (comedian, actor, film director)
1940 Richard Pryor (actor)
1945 Bette Midler (actress, singer)

Famous People born on December 2nd
1946 Gianni Versace (fashion designer)
1973 Monica Seles (tennis player)
1981 Britney Spears (singer)

Famous People born on December 3rd
1930 Jean-Luc Godard (film director)
1948 Ozzy Osbourne (singer)

Famous People born on December 4th
1892 Francisco Franco (Spanish dictator)
1949 Jeff Bridges (actor)

1964 Marisa Tomei (actress)

Famous People born on December 5th

1782 Martin Van Buren (8th US President)
1839 George Armstrong Custer (US General)
1901 Walt Disney (cartoonist)
1932 Little Richard (singer)

Famous People born on December 6th

1896 Ira Gershwin (musician, lyricist)
1920 Dave Brubeck (musician)

Famous People born on December 7th

1928 Noam Chomsky (linguist, author, political activist)

Famous People born on December 8th

1542 Mary Queen of Scots (British royal)
1925 Sammy Davis Jr. (actor, singer, entertainer)
1936 David Carradine (actor)
1943 Jim Morrison (singer)
1953 Kim Basinger (actress)
1964 Teri Hatcher (actress)
1966 Sinead O'Connor (singer)

Famous People born on December 9th

1608 John Milton (poet)
1916 Kirk Douglas (actor)
1957 Donny Osmond (singer)

Famous People born on December 10th

1830 Emily Dickinson (poet)
1952 Susan Dey (actress)

Famous People born on December 11th

1942 Donna Mills (actress)
1949 Teri Garr (actress)

Famous People born on December 12th

1893 Edward G. Robinson (actor)
1915 Frank Sinatra (singer, actor)

Famous People born on December 13th

1925 Dick Van Dyke (actor)
1948 Ted Nugent (singer)

Famous People born on December 14th

1503 Nostradamus (mystic)
1935 Lee Remick (actress)

Famous People born on December 15th

1892 J. Paul Getty (oil magnate)
1949 Don Johnson (actor)

Famous People born on December 16th

1770 Ludwig Van Beethoven (composer)
1917 Arthur C. Clarke (author, visionary)

Famous People born on December 17th

1797 Joseph Henry (weather scientist)

Famous People born on December 18th

1886 Ty Cobb (baseball player)
1916 Betty Grable (actress)
1943 Keith Richards (musician)
1947 Steven Spielberg (film director)
1963 Brad Pitt (actor)
1980 Christina Aguilera (singer)

Famous People born on December 19th

1915 Edith Piaf (singer, actress)
1972 Alyssa Milano (actress)

Famous People born on December 20th

1946 Uri Geller (magician)
1952 Jenny Agutter (actress)

Famous People born on December 21st

1879 Joseph Stalin (Soviet leader)
1935 Phil Donahue (TV presenter)
1937 Jane Fonda (actress)
1940 Frank Zappa (musician)
1954 Chris Evert (tennis player)

Famous People born on December 22nd

1858 Giacomo Puccini (musician, composer)
1949 Robin Gibb (singer)
1949 Maurice Gibb (singer)

Famous People born on December 23rd

1870 John Marin (artist)
1964 Eddie Veder (singer)

Famous People born on December 24th

1905 Howard Hughes (industrialist)
1922 Ava Gardner (actress)
1971 Ricky Martin (singer)

Famous People born on December 25th

1642 Sir Isaac Newton (scientist)
1887 Conrad Hilton (hotelier)
1899 Humphrey Bogart (actor)
1918 Anwar Sadat (Egyptian President)
1949 Sissy Spacek (actress)
1954 Annie Lennox (singer)
1971 Dido (singer)

Famous People born on December 26th

1791 Charles Babbage (inventor)
1893 Mao Tse-tung (Chinese premier)
1914 Richard Widmark (actor)

Famous People born on December 27th

1571 Johannes Kepler (astronomer, mathematician, scientist, author of the first science fiction novel "Somnium")
1822 Louis Pasteur (scientist)
1901 Marlene Dietrich (singer, actress)
1948 Gerard Depardieu (actor)

Famous People born on December 28th

1856 Woodrow Wilson (28th US President)
1954 Denzel Washington (actor)

Famous People born on December 29th

1808 Andrew Johnson (17th US President)
1936 Mary Tyler Moore (actress)
1938 Jon Voight (actor)
1972 Jude Law (actor)

Famous People born on December 30th

1865 Rudyard Kipling (author)
1928 Bo Diddley (singer)
1945 Davy Jones (singer)
1959 Tracey Ullman (actress, comedienne, singer)
1975 Tiger Woods (golfer)

Famous People born on December 31st

1869 Henri Matisse (artist)
1937 Anthony Hopkins (actor)
1943 Ben Kingsley (actor)
1943 John Denver (singer)
1959 Val Kilmer (actor)

Female Baby Names with Meanings and Origins

African Female Baby Names

Name	Origin	Meaning	Similiar Names
Aba	African	Born on Thursday	
Abeni	African	Girl prayed for	
Abiba	African	Child born after grandmother died	
Aissa	African	Grateful	Izza, Isa, Issa, Asa
Arziki	African Hausa	Prosperity	
Asha	Hindu, African	Hope, life	
Baako	African	First born	
Caimile	African	Name from a proverb	
Catava	African	Bame from a proverb	
Chipo	African	Gift	Chip
Ebere	African	Mercy	
Faizah	African	Victorious	
Femi	African	Love me	
Fola	African	Honour	
Habika	African	Sweetheart	
Halima	African	Gentle	
Isoke	African	Satisfying gift	
Jendayi	African	Give thanks	
Kadija	African	The Prophet's wife	Kadee
Kambo	African	Must work for everything	
Kanene	African	A little thing in the eye is big	

Kapera	African	This child, too, will die	
Karimah	African	Generous	
Kasinda	African	Born to a family with twins	
Keisha	African	Favourite	
Kesia	African	Favourite	
Lateefah	North African	Gentle, pleasant	Latifa, Latiffa, Lateefa
Limber	African	Joyfulness	
Maizah	African	Discerning	
Malika	African	Queen, princess	
Mandisa	African	Sweet	
Marjani	African	Coral	
Nabelung	African	Beautiful one	
Nailah	African	Succeeding	
Narkeasha	African	Pretty	Nar, Keash, Keasha, Kisha
Pemba	African	The force of present existence	
Rashida	African	Righteous	
Raziya	African	Agreeable	
Safiya	African	Pure	
Saidah	African	Happy, fortunate	
Salihah	African	Correct	
Shasmecka	African	Princess	Shas
Sibongile	African	Thanks	
Sitembile	African	Trust	
Sukutai	African	Hug	
Takiyah	North African	Pious, righteous	
Tale	African	Green	
Tapanga	African, Hebrew	Sweet, unpredictable	Tata, Pangi
Zalika	African	Well born	
Zarina	African	Golden	
Zina	African	Name	

Anglo-Saxon Female Baby Names

Name	Origin	Meaning	Similiar Names
Alodie	Anglo-Saxon	Wealthy	
Bliss	Anglo-Saxon	Joy	
Capri	Anglo-Saxon	The goat	
Darlene	Anglo-Saxon	Tenderly beloved, little darling	Darlin, Darlen, Darleen, Darlynn, Dare, Darla
Ebba	Germanic/Anglo-Saxon	Strength, return of the tide	
Faina	Anglo-Saxon	Joyful	
Githa	Anglo-Saxon	Gift	
Kendra	Anglo-Saxon	Knowledge	
Kirby	Anglo-Saxon	From the church town	
Lynn	Anglo-Saxon	A cascade	
Mildred	Anglo-Saxon	Mild, power	Mildrid, Mildraed, Mildryd, Milly, Milli, Milley, Millie, Hildred, Hil, Mil
Walburga	Anglo-Saxon	A mighty defender, a fortress	Walburg

Arabic Female Baby Names

Name	Origin	Meaning	Similiar Names
Aaliyah	Arabic, Hebrew	High exalted, to ascend	Aleah, Alea, Aleaseya, Aliya, Alia, Aleeya, Aliyah, Allyiah
Abia	Arabic	Great	
Adalia	Hebrew, Arabic, German	Refuge of God, just, noble one	
Adara	Greek, Arabic	Beauty, virgin	
Adiva	Arabic	Pleasant, gentle	
Aida	Old English, Arabic	Joyful, helper, reward	
Aiesha	Arabic	Woman	
Ain	Arabic	Precious, eye	
Akilah	Arabic	Intelligent, logical	
Alima	Arabic	Wise, learned	
Alzena	Arabic	The woman	
Amber	Arabic	Yellow-brown, precious jewel	Ambert
Ameerah	Arabic	Princess	Amira, Almira, Allihmyir, Almaia, Alimaia, Almaye
Anan	Arabic	Clouds	
Anisa	Arabic	Friendly	Anissa
Atifa	Arabic	Affection	
Azalea	Arabic	Democracy	
Banan	Arabic	Fingertips	
Barakah	Arabic	White one	
Basimah	Arabic	Smiling	
Beulah	Arabic	Married	
Cala	Arabic	Castle	
Cantara	Arabic	Small bridge	

Carna	Arabic	Horn	
Fatima	Arabic	Daughter of Muhammad	Fatma
Fatin	Arabic	Captivating	
Hadiya	Arabic	Guide to righteousness, gift	
Haifa	Arabic	Slender	Hayfa
Hanan	Arabic	Mercy	
Hasna	Arabic	Beautiful	
Iman	Arabic	Faith, belief	Imani
Israt	Arabic	Affection	Ishrat
Jala	Arabic	Charity	
Jamilah	Arabic	Beautiful	
Jana	Czech, Arabic	God's gracious gift; a harvest of fruit	
Jehan	Arabic	Beautiful flower	
Kalila	Arabic	Beloved	Khalila
Kamilah	Arabic	The perfect one	Camilla, Kamilla
Karida	Arabic	Untouched, virginal	
Khalidah	Arabic	Immortal	
Leila	Arabic	Dark as the night	Lila, Lillah, Lyla, Leilia, Lela, Laila, Layla
Lila	Arabic	Night	
Lina	Arabic	Tender	
Mahala	Native American, Hebrew, Arabic	Woman; tenderness;	Mahalah, Mahalar, Mahela, Mahalia, Mahelia, Mehala
Martha	Arabic	A lady	Marth, Marta, Martina, Marella, Martita, Marti, Marty, Mattie, Matty, Marthe, Masia
Matana	Arabic	Gift	
Myiesha	Arabic	Life's blessing	
Nafeeza	Arabic	Precious thing	Nafiza, Naf, Naffy, Naffo

Naimah	Arabic	Living a soft, enjoyable life	
Nazirah	Arabic	Equal, like	
Nimah	Arabic	Blessing, loan	
Noya	Arabic	Beautiful, ornamented	
Qamra	Arabic	Moon	
Rihana	Arabic	Sweet basil	
Sabirah	Arabic	Patient	
Sabra	Arabic, Hebrew	Thorny cactus; to rest	
Sadira	Arabic	Ostrich returning from water	
Sahara	Arabic	The moon	Shahar
Saida	Arabic	Fortunate one	
Sakinah	Arabic	God-inspired peace-of-mind, tranquility	Sakina
Salimah	Arabic	Safe, healthy	
Salwa	Arabic	Solace; comfort	Salva
Samirah	Arabic	Entertaining companion	
Samma	Arabic	Sky,	Sa, Samm, Ma
Saree	Arabic	Most noble	
Selima	Arabic	Peace	Selin
Shakira	Arabic	Grateful	
Shammara	Arabic	He girded his loins	
Siham	Arabic	Arrows	
Sumehra	Arabic	Beautiful face	
Summer	Old English, Arabic	Summer season	Sumar, Somar, Samar
Tahirah	Arabic	Chaste, pure	
Thana	Arabic	Gratitude	
Thara	Arabic	Wealth	
Vega	Arabic	Falling star	
Widjan	Arabic	Ecstacy	
Xaviera	Arabic, Basque	Bright, new house	Xavière
Zahara	Arabic	Shining, luminous	
Zahra	Arabic, Swahili	White, flowers	
Zaida	Arabic	Fortunate one	
Zaira	Arabic	Rose	Zahirah, Zaire, Zi, Zizi
Zara	Hebrew, Arabic	Dawn, princess	Zarah, Zarry, Zari, Zerlinda
Zaria	Arabic	Rose	Zariah, Zari

Zaza	Hebrew, Arabic	Movement, flowery	
Zuleika	Arabic	Fair-haired	Zuleyka

Armenian Female Baby Names

Name	Origin	Meaning	Similiar Names
Anahid	Armenian	Goddess of the Moon	
Anoush	Armenian	Sweet	
Araxie	Armenian	River said to inspire poetic expression	
Carine	Armenian	Friend	
Dikranouhi	Armenian	Queen	
Karyan	Armenian	The dark one	
Lucine	Armenian	Moon	
Ohanna	Armenian	God's gracious gift	
Perouze	Armenian	Turquoise	
Siran	Armenian	Alluring	
Siroun	Armenian	Lovely	
Ziazan	Armenian	Rainbow	

Basque Female Baby Names

Name	Origin	Meaning	Similiar Names
Amaia	Basque	End	
Aurkene	Basque	Presentation	
Bakarne	Basque	Solitude	
Deiene	Basque	Religious holiday	
Gizane	Basque	Christ's incarnation	
Gotzone	Basque	Angel, messenger	
Iratze	Basque	In reference to the Virgin Mary	
Jaione	Basque	Nativity	
Jakinda	Basque	Hyacinth	
Kepa	Basque	Stone	
Lore	Basque	A flower	
Xaviera	Arabic, Basque	Bright, new house	Xavière

Celtic Female Baby Names

Name	Origin	Meaning	Similiar Names
Africa	Celtic	Pleasing, pleasant	Affrica
Aileen	Greek, Celtic	Light, green meadow	Leener, Leen
Aine	Celtic	Joy	
Aislinn	Celtic	A dream, vision, inspiration	Aisling
Aithne	Celtic	Lttle fire	
Arlene	Celtic	Pledge	Arleen, Arline, Arlette, Arlynn, Arlyn, Arleine, Arlen
Birkita	Celtic	Strength	
Bree	Celtic	Broth	
Brenna	Celtic	Raven maid, dark-haired	
Bretta	Celtic	From	Brette
Briana	Celtic	Strong	Brianne, Brianna, Breanna
Bridget	Celtic	Resolute, strength, saint	Brigetta, Brigette, Brigitte, Brighid, Brigid, Britta, Brita, Britte, Brit, Biddy, Brie, Bree, Birgit, Birgitta, Brigada, Brigida, Brigita, Birgit, Birdie, Bryde, Bridge, Gidget, Gidgey
Brietta	Celtic	Strong	
Brina	Celtic	Protector	
Brites	Celtic	Strength	Britta
Caitlin	Celtic, Welsh	Pure	Caitlyn, Kaitlin, Kaitlyn, Katelyn, Catelyn, Caitrin

Caoimhe	Celtic	Gentleness, beauty, grace	
Cerdwin	Celtic	The Mother Goddess	
Colleen	Celtic, Gaelic	Girl	Colene, Coleen
Cordelia	Latin, Celtic	Rope, heart, a sea jewel	Delia, Cordy, Kordelia
Cuyler	Celtic	Chapel	
Dana	Swedish, Celtic	From Denmark, Mother of the Gods in myths	
Devnet	Celtic	poet	
Dierdre	Celtic	Young girl, one who rages, broken-hearted	Deirdre, Deirdra, Dierdra, Deedee, Deedra, Dee
Edana	Celtic	Zealous, fiery	
Eilis	Hebrew, Celtic	God's oath	
Erin	Celtic/Gaelic	Peace, western island	Errin, Erinne, Eryn, Erynn, Erinna, Erynna
Erlina	Celtic	Girl from Ireland	
Etain	Celtic	Shining	
Evelyn	Celtic	Lively, pleasant	Eileen, Eilen, Ilene, Alene, Eveline, Evalyn, Aveline, Avaline, Avelina, Avalina, Evel, Evilio, Evalina, Evelina, Evette
Fainche	Celtic	Saint's name	
Fallon	Celtic	Grandchild of the ruler, in charge	
Fiona	Celtic	White, fair	Fione, Fionnula
Gilda	Celtic	God's servent	
Gwendolyn	Celtic	White brow	Gwendolynne, Gwendoline
Isolde	Celtic	Beautiful	
Kaie	Celtic	Combat	

Kaitlyn	Celtic	Little darling	Kaitlin, Kaitlynne, Kait, Katie, Kaydee, Katlan
Kathleen	Celtic	Little darling	Caitlin
Keelin	Celtic	Slender, fair	
Lindsay	Old English, Celtic	Pool island; linden island	Lindsey, Lyndsay, Lyndsey, Lyndsy, Lynsey, Linsey, Lindy, Lindzee
Lorna	Celtic	of Lorne	
Moira	Irish, Celtic	Bitter; great	Maura, Moyra
Morgance	Celtic	Sea-dweller	
Morgandy	Celtic	Little one from the edge of the sea	
Pixie	Celtic	Small elf, faery	Pixy, Pixi, Piksi, Piksy
Rhonda	Celtic	Good spear	
Saraid	Celtic	Excellent	
Seanna	Celtic	God's grace	Shawna, Shawny, Shawnie, Shawnna, Shaune, Shauna, Siana, Shay
Shayla	Celtic	Fairy palace	
Shela	Celtic	Musical	
Shylah	Celtic	Loyal to God, strong	Shy, Shyla
Tara	Celtic, Gaelic, Hindu	Rocky hill, tower	Taria, Taryn
Treasa	Celtic	Strong	
Treva	Celtic	Prudent	Treve
Tully	Celtic, Gaelic	A people, peaceful one	
Ula	Celtic, Old German	Sea jewel, inherited estate	

Chinese Female Baby Names

Name	Origin	Meaning	Similiar Names
An	Chinese	Peace	
Chyou	Chinese	Autumn	
Genji	Chinese	Gold	
Jun	Chinese	Truth	
Lian	Chinese	The graceful willow	
Lien	Chinese	Lotus	
Mingmei	Chinese	Smart, beautiful	Mingmey

Czech Female Baby Names

Name	Origin	Meaning	Similiar Names
Anezka	Czech	Pure	
Bela	Czech	White	
Beta	Czech	Dedicated to God	
Dita	Czech	Rich gift	
Eliska	Czech	Truthful	
Jana	Czech, Arabic	God's gracious gift; a harvest of fruit	
Marjeta	Czech	Pearl	
Nadezda	Czech	One with hope	
Ryba	Czech	Fish	
Zdenka	Czech	One from Sidon, a winding sheet	
Zelenka	Czech	Little innocent one	
Zuza	Czech	Graceful	

Danish Female Baby Names

Name	Origin	Meaning	Similiar Names
Aslog	Danish	Consecrated to God	
Astrid	Danish	Beautiful Goddess	
Benedikte	Danish	Blessed	Bemte
Berit	Danish	High Goddess	
Bine	Danish	Supplanter, Representative	
Dagmar	Danish	Joy day, bright	
Grette	Danish	Pearl	
Saffi	Danish	Wisdom	
Silje	Danish	Blind	
Sofie	Danish	Wise	
Solovej	Danish	Strong Home	
Tordis	Danish	Thor's Goddess	
Trine	Danish	Blessed , Pure, Holy	
Ulf	Danish	Wolf	
Ulrike	Danish	Powerful , Prosperous	
Vibeke	Danish	War	
Vita	Danish	Life	

Dutch Female Baby Names

Name	Origin	Meaning	Similiar Names
Aledis	Dutch	Noble, Kind	
Anneke	Dutch	Gracious	Annemarie, Annika, Annikalyn, Anouk, Antje, Annikalyn
Brandy	Dutch	Brandy, Warm and Comforting Drink	
Cokkie	Dutch	Yellow Colored, Horn	
Dorothea	Dutch	Gift Of God	
Elke	Dutch	Noble, Kind	
Femke	Dutch	Girl	
Fenna	Dutch	White, Fair	
Georgina	Dutch	Farmer	
Gerda	Dutch	Penn	
Gertunde	Dutch	Strong Spear	
Gilberta	Dutch	Bright Pledge	
Gisela	Dutch	Pledge	
Greet	Dutch	Pearl	Greetje, Gretje
Hadewych	Dutch	War, Strife	
Heike	Dutch	Ruler of the Home	
Hilda	Dutch	Battle	
Isabella	Dutch	Consecrated to God	Lisabeth, Liseje, Lijsbeth, Lisanne
Jacintha	Dutch	Hyacinth	
Janneke	Dutch	Gos is Gracious	Jahanneke
Kaatje	Dutch	Pure	
Katrien	Dutch	Blessed, Pure, Holy	
Kort	Dutch	Bold, Wise Counselor	
Kunigonde	Dutch	Brave Warrior	
Kyler	Dutch	Archer	

Libel	Dutch	Dragonfly	

Egyptian Female Baby Names

Name	Origin	Meaning	Similiar Names
Amarna	Egyptian	Reformed	
Chione	Egyptian	Daughter of Nile	
Isis	Egyptian	Mythical Goddess of Sky and Nature	
Lapis	Egyptian	Jewel	
Mariasha	Egyptian	Perfect	
Mauli	Egyptian	Black	
Memphis	Egyptian	Good Place to Live	
Menefer	Egyptian	Beautiful City	
Montsho	Egyptian	Mountain	
Mry	Egyptian	Loved	
Myrrh	Egyptian	Natural Scent	
Neith	Egyptian	Divine Mother	
Nenet	Egyptian	Water Goddess	
Nile	Egyptian	From the River Nile	
Nubia	Egyptian	From Nubia	
Sahirah	Egyptian	Clean, Pristine	
Sanura	Egyptian	Kitten	
Tauret	Egyptian	Pregnant Women Goddess	
Yanara	Egyptian	Shining Light	

English Female Baby Names

Name	Origin	Meaning	Similiar Names
Afton	Old English	River name	Aftonio
Aida	Old English, Arabic	Joyful, helper, reward	
Aldercy	Old English	A chief	
Amaris	English	Child of the moon	
Ashley	Old English	Ash-tree	Ashleigh, Ashford, Ash, Ashe, Ashby, Ashlan, Ashlie, Ashling, Ashlyn, Ashlin, Ashli, Ashi
Audrey	Old English	Noble strength	Audry, Audery, Audra, Audey, Audie
Avena	English	Oats	
Blossom	Old English	Lovely	
Blythe	Old English	Joyous	Blithe
Brenda	Old English, German	Fiery hill, sword-blade	Brynna, Brynn, Brenunda
Brook	Old English	Stream	Brooke, Brooks, Brookes
Bunny	English	Little rabbit	
Burdette	Middle English	Small bird	
Carling	Old English	Hill where old women or witches gather	
Chelsea	Old English	River landing place, port	Chelsie, Kelsie, Kelsey, Kelsy
Claiborne	Old English	Born of the earth	Clayborne, Claybourne, Claibourne, Clayton, Clay
Clovis	Old English	Clover	Clothilde, Clotilde
Columbia	Old English	A dove	
Corliss	Old English	Cheerful and generous	

Courtney	Old English, French	From the court	Cortney, Cortie, Corey, Court, Kurt, Kurtney, Kort, Kortney
Daisy	Latin, Old English	Day's eye, flower name	Daisey
Daralis	Old English	Beloved	
Dawn	Old English	Dawn	
Deanna	Latin, Old English	Valley	Deane, Deanna, Deana, Deanne, Deena
Demelza	Old English	Fort on a hill	Demie
Devon	Old English	Defender	Devin
Dooriya	English	The sea	
Dory	English	Golden-haired	
Eartha	Old English	Of the earth	
Easter	Old English	Easter time	
Ebony	English/Greek	Dark beauty, a hard wood	Ebonie, Ebonee
Edda	Old English	Rich	Eda
Edlyn	Old English	Noble woman	
Edolie	Old English	Boble	
Edsel	Old English	Rich	
Ella	Old English/Old German	Beautiful fairy woman	Ellie
Ember	Old English	Smoldering remains of a fire	
Ena	Old English	Wife, soul	Enna
Erika	Old Norse, Old English, Old German	Ever-powerful	Erica, Eryka, Ericka, Enrica
Farrah	English, Latin	Beautiful, wild ass	Farah, Farra
Fern	Old English	Leafy plant	Ferne, Fearn, Fearne, Fernly
Fleta	Old English	Swift, fleet	
Gail	Old English	Gay, lively	Gayle, Gale
Gaines	Middle English	Increase in wealth	Gaynes, Gainsborough, Gainor, Gaynor
Gleda	Old English	To make happy	
Goldie	Old English	Gold	
Gypsy	Old English	Wanderer	

Gytha	Old English	A gift	
Harmony	English	A beautiful blending	
Harva	Old English	Army warrior	Harvelle, Harvina, Harvine
Haylee	Old English	From the hay meadow	Hayleigh, Hayley
Hazel	Old English	Commander	
Heather	Old English	Heather	
Holly	Old English	Plant with red berries, holly grove	Holli, Hollie, Hollee, Hollye
Honey	Old English	Honey	
Hope	English	Trust, faith	
Ida	Old English	Prosperous	
India	Sanskrit, English	River; from India	
Jillian	Old English	Girl	Jill
Joy	Old English	Joy	Joie, Joia, Gioa
Kaelyn	Old English	Meadow	
Kirsten	Greek, Old English	Christian; stone church	Kristine, Kristi, Kirstin, Kirstie, Kirsty, Kirsti, Kiersten, Kier
Kismet	English	Fate, destiny	
Kyla	Gaelic, Old English	Narrow, narrow channel, honor	Kylene, Kylee, Ky
Lainey	English	Sun ray	Laine
Lari	English	Crowned with laurel	
Lark	English	A bird	Larkin, Lirkin
Leigh	Old English	Meadow	
Leslie	Scottish, Old English	Dweller in the gray castle; small meadow	Lesley, Lesly, Les, Lee
Liberty	English	Freedom	Libby,
Lindsay	Old English, Celtic	Pool island; linden island	Lindsey, Lyndsay, Lyndsey, Lyndsy, Lynsey, Linsey, Lindy, Lindzee
Locke	Old English	Stronghold	
Love	Old English	Loved one	Lovie

Luella	Old English	Elfin	Louella, Loella, Luelle
Maida	Old English	A maiden	Maidie, Maidy, Mady, Maidel, Mayda
Maitane	Old English	Beloved	
Mala	Old French, Old English	Bad one; meeting hall	
Manhattan	Old English, Scottish	Whiskey	Manny, Manda, Maisie
Mercy	Middle English	Compassion, pity	Merci, Mercia
Merry	Middle English	Joyful	Merri, Merrie, Merrilee, Merrily, Merrita, Merrielle
Missy	Old English	Young girl	Missie, Missye, Sissy
Misty	Old English	Covered by mist	Mistee
Nara	Old English, Gaelic, Native American	Near one; joyous; place name	
Neda	Slavic, English	Born on Sunday; sanctuary	Nedda, Neddy, Ned, Nerida, Nedjelko, Nedo
Palma	Old English	Palm bearing pilgrim	Palmyra, Palmira, Palmiera
Pearl	Middle English	Gemstone	Pearla, Perle, Pearle, Perla, Purlie, Pegeen
Pebbles	English	A stone	
Poppy	Old English	Flower	
Queena	Old English	Queen	
Quella	English	Pacify	
Radella	Old English	Elfin advisor	
Richelle	Old German, Old English	Powerful ruler; brave one	Ricarda, Ricky, Rikki

Roberta	Old English	Bright, famous	Ruperta, Robin, Robyn, Robbin, Robinette, Robina, Bobbi, Bobbie, Bobby, Bert, Berta, Bertie, Berthe
Rowena	Gaelic, Old English	Red-haired; rugged	Rowana
Rumer	English	Gypsy	
Ryesen	English	Rye	
Salal	English	A plant	
Saxon	Latin, English	Large stone; swordsman	
Scarlet	Middle English	Deep red	Scarlett
Selby	Old English	Of the manor house farm	Selden, Seldon, Selwin, Selwyn
Shandy	Old English	Rambunctious	
Sharman	English	A fair share	
Shelby	English	Sheltered town	
Shirley	Old English	Country meadow	Shirlee, Sherlie, Shurlie, Shirleigh, Shirleen, Sherey, Shirl, Shurl, Shir
Skyla	English	Sky, sheltering	Sky
Skylar	English	Eternal life, strength, love and beauty	Skye, Sky, Skyrah
Sparrow	English	A bird	
Spring	English	Spring season	
Stockard	English	From the yard of tree stumps	
Storm	Old English	Stormy weather, tempest	Storme, Stormy, Stormie
Summer	Old English, Arabic	Summer season	Sumar, Somar, Samar
Tatum	Old English	Cheerful bringer of joy	Tait, Taitum, Tat, Tayte, Taite

Tavia	Latin, Old English	Great	Tay, Taves, Tay
Tawnie	English	Little one, yellowish-brown	Tawny
Thistle	Old English	Thistle	
Tina	Old English, Hindu	River	Tyna
Trudy	Old English	Beloved	
Tuesday	Old English	The day of the week	
Ulla	Old English	To fill up	
Ulrika	Old German, Old English	Wolf ruler	Ulrica, Ulrike
Vala	Old English	Chosen	
Velvet	Middle English	Fabric	
Verity	English	Verity, truth	Verita
Wendy	Old English	Fair	
Whitney	Old English	From the white island	
Willow	Middle English	Freedom, tree	
Wilona	Old English	Desired	
Yedda	Old English	Singing	Yetta
Zinnia	English	Flower name	Zinia, Zin, Zina

French Female Baby Names

Name	Origin	Meaning	Similiar Names
Adora	French	Beloved one	
Alavda	French	Lark	
Amarante	French	Flower name	
Angevin	French	Angel of wine	Angie, Angel, Angelus
Aubrey	German, Old French	Elf rule	
Babette	French	Stranger,lovely	Elizabeth
Bedelia	French	Strength	
Belle	French	Beautiful	Bella, Belva
Berangèr	French	Courage of a bear	
Bonamy	French	Good friend	
Brie	French	Region in France	
Brier	French	Heather	
Caresse	French	Beloved	
Caron	French	Pure	
Chanel	French	Canal	
Chantal	French	A song, stony place	
Charlotte	French	Petite and feminine	Charlie, Carlotta, Lottie, Lotte, Charlene, Charmaine, Charmayne, Charlayne, Chatzie
Cheryl	French	Beloved, dear	Sherryl, Sherryll, Sherrill, Sheryl, Cheryle, Sheryle, Cher, Cherrie, Cherry, Cherish, Cheri, Cherie, Sheri,

			Sherry
Courtney	Old English, French	From the court	Cortney, Cortie, Corey, Court, Kurt, Kurtney, Kort
Crescent	Old French	One who creates	
Cyprien	French	Cypriot	
Dacio	French	From arcy	
Deja	French	Before	Dejah
Demi	French	Half, small	
Desiree	Latin, French	So long hoped for, crave, desire	Desi, Desideria, Desirae, Desiri
Destinee	French	Destiny	Desi, Des, Destini, Destiny
Destry	French	War horse	
Diamanta	French	Like a diamond	
Doreen	French	Golden	Dorene, Dorine
Elaine	Old French	Light	Elaina, Elayne, Elana, Alaine, Alana, Laine, Laney
Elita	French	Special one	
Elle	French	Woman, girl	
Eloise	French	Intelligent, smart	Elouise, Elo, El
Fantine	French	Childlike	
Fawne	Old French, Latin	Young deer	Fawn, Faun, Fauna, Fawna
Faye	French	Fairy	Fay, Fey
Fayme	French	Held in high esteem	
Felicite	French	Fortunate	

Frances	Latin, Old French	From France, free	Fanchon, Francesca, Fran, Franny, Fanny, Frannie, Francine, Franchesca
Geneva	Old French	Juniper berry	Genevia, Genny
Genevieve	French	White wave	Genny
Ghislaine	French	Sweet pledge	
Iolanthe	French	Violet	
Jaimie	French	I love	
Jamari	French	Warrior	
Jenay	French	Name of a plant	Jenai
Jolie	French	Pretty, merry	
Lacy	French	Place name	Lacey, Laycee, Lace
Laverne	Old French	From the alder grove, spring-like	La Verne, Verna, Verne, Lally
Leala	French	Loyal one	
Liana	French, Latin	Vine, to bind; youth	Lianna, Lianne, Liane, Leana
Linette	Middle French	Linnet bird, flaxen	Linnette, Lynette, Linnet, Linetta, Linn
Mabel	French, Latin	My fair maid; lovely	Maybelle, Mabel, Maibelle, Mabella, Maybelline, Mabry, Amabel
Magnolia	French	A flower	
Mala	Old French, Old English	Bad one; meeting hall	
Mallory	French	Mailed	

Marcella	Latin, French	God of war; little hammer	Marcy, Marcie, Marcelle, Marceline, Marclyn, Marcelin, Marciana
Marianne	Old French	Little Mary	Manya , Marianna, Mara, Marian, Marisha, Marilyn, Maire, Marion, Marrion, Mariana, Mariann, Mary-Ann, Maryanne
Marjorie	Old French	Pearl	Marjory, Marjorey, Marjary, Margery, Margey, Margie, Marge, Margo, Marje, Marjy, Marcail
Marvelle	Old French	Miracle	Marvel, Marvell, Marva, Marvella
Maureen	Latin, Gaelic, Old French	Great; little Mary; dark-haired	May, Maura, Mora, Moira, Moreen, Moria, Moriah, Maurin, Maurine, Morena, Maurizia, Mo
Mignon	French	Dainty, petite	
Montague	French	Steep mountain	Montagu,

			Montag
Musetta	Old French	A ballad	Musette, Musa, Muse
Myra	Latin, French	Wonderful; quiet song	
Noella	French	Christmas	Noelle
Odetta	French	Melody	
Odette	French	Happy home	
Olive	Old Norse, Latin, Old French	Kind one; olive tree, peace	Olivia, Olivya, Olivette, Ollie, Olly, Olva, Livia, Livy, Liv, Livvy, Nollie, Nola
Orane	French	Rising	
Oriel	Old French	Golden, angel of destiny	Orielle
Pansy	French	Thought	Pansee, Pansie, Pense
Papillon	French	Butterfly	
Pascale	French	Born at Easter	
Purvis	French	Provide	
Quiterie	French	Tranquil	
Raissa	Old French, Greek	Thinker; rose	Raisa
Remy	French	From Rheims	
Riva	French	River	Rivy, Reeva, Rive, Rivi, Ria, Reva
Rochelle	French	From the little rock	Rochella, Rochette
Roslin	Old French	Little red-haired one	Rosselin, Roslyn, Rose-Lynn, Rosalyn, Rosalind, Rosalinde, Rosalinda, Rosalynda
Ruby	Old French	Red gem	Rubie, Rubee, Rubia, Rubina
Salina	Latin, French	By the salt water; solemn	Saleena
Searlait	French	Petite	

Sennett	French	Wise one	Senet, Senta
Shannelle	French	Channel	Chanel, Shanel, Schannel, Channel, Shannel, Shanelly
Shantay	French	Enchanted	
Shantelle	French		Telle, Telly, Shanty
Sigourney	French	Daring king	
Solange	French	Rare jewel	
Soleil	French	Sun	
Sydney	Old French	From city of St. Denis	Sidney, Sydny, Sid, Sidne, Sidoney, Sidonia, Siddie, Syd, Sydell, Sidell, Sydel
Tayce	French	Silence	
Taylar	Old French	To cut	Tayla
Tempest	Old French	Storm	Tempestt
Tiffany	Old French	Appearance of God	Tiff, Tifany, Tiphany, Tifanee, Tiffy, Tiffie, Fanny
Tracy	French	Path, road	Tracey
Troy	French	Place name	
Vail	Old French	From the valley	Vayle, Vale, Valle, Val
Valerie	Old French, Latin	Valor, strong	Valeria, Valery, Valerian, Vally, Vallie, Val, Valarie, Vallerie

Gaelic Female Baby Names

Name	Origin	Meaning	Similiar Names
Alana	Gaelic, Hawaiian	Fair, beautiful, offering	Alaina, Alyn, Allyn, Lani, Allie, Ally, Alli, Lanny, Alun, Alanna, Laina, Lane, Laney, Elaine, Alona
Apirka	Gaelic	Pleasant	
Caley	Gaelic	Slender	
Cayleigh	Gaelic	Party	Cay, Lee, Leigh, Caylah
Colleen	Celtic, Gaelic	Girl	Colene, Coleen
Dacey	Gaelic	Southerner	
Darby	Gaelic	Free man	Derby
Darcy	Gaelic	Dark	D'Arcy, Darcie, Darcey, Darci
Darra	Gaelic, Farsi	Small great one, riches	Dara
Decla	Gaelic	Goodness	
Delaney	Gaelic	Descendant of the challenger	Delaina, Delaine
Dymphna	Gaelic	Suitable one, virgin saint	
Erin	Celtic/Gaelic	Peace, western island	Errin, Erinne, Eryn, Erynn, Erinna, Erynna

Fennella	Gaelic	White shoulder	Finola
Glenna	Gaelic	From the valley	
Grania	Gaelic	Love	Grainne
Keely	Gaelic	Beautiful and graceful	Keeley, Kealy, Keel, Keelan, Keeler
Kellan	Gaelic	Warrior princess	
Kelly	Gaelic, Teutonic	Church, warrior, wood, holly; farm by the spring	Kel
Kennis	Gaelic	Beautiful	
Kyla	Gaelic, Old English	Narrow, narrow channel, honor	Kylene, Kylee, Ky
Kyna	Gaelic	Wise	Kyne, Cyna, Cyne
Mab	Gaelic	Joy	Mave, Mavis, Mabley
Malvina	Gaelic	Smooth snow	Malva, Malvie, Melvina, Melvine, Mevin, Mally, Melly, Mal, Mel, Mellen
Maureen	Latin, Gaelic, Old French	Great; little Mary; dark-haired	May, Maura, Mora, Moira, Moreen, Moria, Moriah, Maurin, Maurine, Morena, Maurizia, Mo
Meara	Gaelic	Merry	Mira, Meera
Meckenzie	Gaelic	Daughter of the Wise Leader	

Megan	Greek, Gaelic, Welsh	Mighty, strong able, pearl	Meggy, Meghan, Meagan, Megann, Meggy, Meggie, Meg, Megs
Mona	Latin, Greek, Gaelic, Italian	Peaceful; individual; noble one; My lady	
Morgan	Gaelic, Welsh	White sea; bright, dweller by the sea	Morgana, Morganne, Morganica
Myrna	Gaelic	Polite one, gentle	Muirne, Merna, Mirna, Moina, Morna, Moyna
Nara	Old English, Gaelic, Native American	Near one; joyous; place name	
Neala	Gaelic	Champion	Niela, Nela, Neela, Neila, Nealah, Neilla, Nila
Oona	Gaelic, Latin	Unity	Ona, Oonaugh, Oonagh
Rhoswen	Gaelic	White rose	
Riane	Gaelic	Little king	
Rona	Gaelic	Covenant, oath	
Rowena	Gaelic, Old English	Red-haired; rugged	Rowana
Shanley	Gaelic	Child of the old hero	
Sine	Gaelic	God's gracious gift	
Sorcha	Gaelic	Bright	
Tara	Celtic, Gaelic, Hindu	Rocky hill, tower	Taria, Taryn
Tully	Celtic, Gaelic	A people, peaceful one	
Velvia	Gaelic	Woman with a melodious voice	

German Female Baby Names

Name	Origin	Meaning	Similiar Names
Adalgisa	Old German	Noble hostage	Adalgisal, Adelgiese
Adalia	Hebrew, Arabic, German	Refuge of God, just, noble one	
Adelina	Old German	Noble	
Adolfina	German	Noble wolf, noble hero	Adolpha, Adolfa
Agneta	Greek, Germanic	Pure	
Alberta	German	Noble and bright	Albertina, Albertine,
Alice	Old German, Greek	Noble, truth	Alicia, Alise, Alisa, Alison, Allison, Alyse, Alix, Alyce, Alexis, Alika, Aliki, Ali, Allie, Ally, Alisha, Alishea, Alyshia, Alysha, Alissa, Alyson, Alyssa, Allyssa, Al, Lyssa, Alseia, Alessa
Amara	Esperanto, German	Bitter, eternal, immortal, steadfast, beloved	Amarande, Mara
Antje	German	Grace	
Arabelle	German	Beautiful eagle	Arabel, Arabella
Aubrey	German, Old French	Elf rule	
Ava	German	A bird	Avaset
Berit	Old German	Bright, glorious	

Bernadette	German	Bold as a bear	Bern, Bernie, Bernadette, Bernadete, Bernadett, Bernadine, Bernadina
Berta	Germanic, Slavic	Glorious, learning	
Bluma	Old German	A flower, bloom	
Brenda	Old English, German	Fiery hill, sword-blade	Brynna, Brynn, Brenunda
Callan	German	Chatter	Calla
Carleigh	German	Freeholder	
Caroline	Old German	Strong, melody, song	Carolyne, Carolyn, Carolina, Cary, Carly, Carol, Karoline, Karolyne, Karolina, Karolyna, Caro, Karo, Carra, Cara, Carrie, Carry, Lina, Kari, Kerry, Carey, Ceray, Kerrie, Karri, Cary, Karrie, Kerrolyn
Cecania	German	Free	
Chay	Old German	Man	
Chloris	Old German	Pale	Cloris
Clay	German	Adhere, mortal	Clayborne, Clayton, Clayland
Dagmar	Germanic, Danish	Joyous day, bright, joy of the Danes	
Dagna	Old German	A splendid day	
Dame	German	Lady	
Ebba	Germanic/Anglo-	Strength, return of the tide	

	Saxon		
Edwina	German	Prosperous friend, heir's axe	Edina, Edwina, Edwynna, Edwinna, Edwyna
Elisabeth	Hebrew/Germanic	God's oath	Elizabeth, Ellyzabeth, Elise, Elyse, Elysia, Eliza, Beth, Bess, Liz, Lizzy, Elsa, Elsie, Elpeth, Elsbeth, Lisbeth, Lizzie, Liza, Ellie, Bess, Betty, Bette, Bettie, Betsy, Aliza, Arlise, Arlisa, Libby, Isabel, Isabelle, Isabella, Ilse
Ella	Old English/Old German	Beautiful fairy woman, all	Ellie
Emily	Old German/Latin	Industrious, eager	Emilie, Emelie, Emilia, Emelia, Emiline, Emaline, Emmeline, Emmaline, Emyln, Emelyn, Emmilyne, Em
Emma	Old German	Universal, all-embracing	Emmie, Emmy, Em
Erika	Old Norse, Old English, Old German	Ever-powerful	Erica, Eryka, Ericka, Enrica
Ernestine	Old German	Earnest, vigorous	Earnestine, Ernesta, Ernie, Erna

Faiga	Germanic	A bird	
Frederika	Old German	Peaceful ruler	Fredericka, Frederica, Freda, Federica, Friederike
Frieda	Old German	Peace, joy	Friede, Freida, Fredie, Freda, Winifred
Gerda	German	Protection	
Giselle	Old German	A pledge	Gisela
Gretchen	German	Little pearl	
Heidi	German	Noble, kind	
Henrietta	Old German	Ruler of the home	Henriette, Henriella
Idonia	Old German	Industrious	
Jarvia	Old German	Spear-keen	
Jarvinia	German	Keen intelligence	
Jenell	German	Knowledge, understanding, kindness	Jen, Jeni
Leopolda	Old German	Bold leader	Leopoldine
Leyna	Old German	Little angel	Leyns, Lenya
Liese	German	Beloved by God	Liesl, Lieselotte
Lorelei	German	From the Rhine River	
Lorraine	Old German	Where Lothar dwells	Lorry, Lorrie, Loretta, Lorette, Lorne, Lorna, Lori
Louise	Old German	Warrior maiden	Luise, Louisa, Louisiana, Luisa, Loise, Lois, Loyce, Lisette, Luana, Luane, Luwana, Lou, Lu, Lulu, Lulie, Ouise, Ouisa, Eloise, Eloisa, Aloysia, Liusadh

Mallory	Old German	Army counseler, without good fortune	Mallorie, Mallorey, Malori, Malory, Mal, Mally, Malin
Marlene	German	Child of light, bitter	Marlena, Marleen, Marline, Marly, Marlie, Marla, Lene, Lena
Mathilda	Old German	Battle maiden, strength	Matilda, Matelda, Maitilde, Mathylda, Mathilde, Matty, Mattye, Mattie, Maddy, Maddie, Mala, Tila, Tilly, Tillie, Tilda
Maud	Old German	Strength in battle	Maude, Maudie
Millicent	Old German	Industrious, strength	Millisent, Melicent, Milly, Millie, Mili, Melly, Melisande, Melisenda
Minna	Old German, Scottish, Hebrew	Love; mother; bitterness	Mina, Minette, Minetta, Minda, Myna, Mindy
Morgen	German	Morning	
Nixie	Old German	Water sprite	
Norberta	Old German	Blond hero	

Nordica	German	From the north	Norna
Odelia	Old German; Hebrew	Little wealthy one; praise God	Odella, Odelinda, Odilia, Odelette
Olinda	Old German	Protector of property	
Orlantha	Old German	From the land	
Pepin	Old German	Perseverance	Peppy, Pepi, Pippin, Pip, Pippi
Richelle	Old German, Old English	Powerful ruler; brave one	Ricarda, Ricky, Rikki
Roderica	Old German	Famous one	Roderika
Schmetterling	German	Butterfly	
Senta	Old German	Assistant	
Serilda	Old German	Armed maiden of war	
Sonnenschein	German	Sunshine	
Ula	Celtic, Old German	Sea jewel, inherited estate	
Ulrika	Old German, Old English	Wolf ruler	Ulrica, Ulrike
Uta	German	Fortunate maid of battle	Ute
Viveka	German	Little woman, of the strong fortress	
Wanda	Old German	Wanderer	Wenda, Wandis, Wendeline, Wendy, Vanda
Zelda	Old German	Gray warrior	Selda
Zelinda	Old German	Shield of victory	Segelinde

Greek Female Baby Names

Name	Origin	Meaning	Similiar Names
Acacia	Greek	Thorny, naive	Acazia, Acatia
Acantha	Greek	Thorny	
Achlys	Greek	Mist, darknesss	
Adara	Greek, Arabic	Beauty, virgin	
Ademia	Greek	Without husband	
Adonia	Greek	Beautiful	
Adrienne	Greek, Latin	Rich, wealthy, dark one	Adria, Adrea, Adriana, Adrianna, Adrianne, Adreena, Hatria, Adri, Age
Agatha	Greek	Good, kind	Agathe, Agace, Aggie, Aggy, Agata
Aglaia	Greek	Wisdom, glory	Aglaian, Aglai
Agnes	Latin, Greek	Lamb, pure, chaste	Agnese, Agnesa, Aggie, Aggy, Agenta, Inez, Ines, Nessa, Neza, Ynes, Ynez, Annice, Annis
Agneta	Greek, Germanic	Pure	
Aileen	Greek, Celtic	Light, green meadow	Leener, Leen
Airlia	Greek	Ethereal	
Alala	Greek	War goddess	
Alcina	Greek	Strongminded	
Alena	Greek, Slavic	Pretty, light	Olena
Alethea	Greek	Truthful one	

Alice	Old German, Greek	Noble, truth	Alicia, Alise, Alisa, Alison, Allison, Alyse, Alix, Alyce, Alexis, Alika, Aliki, Ali, Allie, Ally, Alisha, Alishea, Alyshia, Alysha, Alissa, Alyson, Alyssa, Allyssa, Al, Lyssa, Alseia, Alessa
Alida	Greek, Latin	Beautiful dressed, small winged one	Aleda, Aletta, Alette, Allida, Allidia, Alidia, Lida
Althea	Greek	Healer, wholesome	Allie, Alethea, Alithea, Thea
Alysa	Greek	Princess	
Alyssa	Greek	Logical	
Amethyst	Greek	A precious stone	
Anastasia	Greek	Resurrection	Anastasio, Anastace, Anastasius, Anastice, Anstasie, Stacia, Stasa, Stacy, Stacey, Natasha, Tasia, Tasha
Andromeda	Greek	Beautiful maiden rescued by Perseus	
Anemone	Greek	Breath, windflower	

Angela	Greek	Heavenly messenger	Angelica, Ange, Angel, Angell, Angie, Anjelica, Angelina, Angelic
Anteia	Greek	Wife of sea-god Proteus	
Anthea	Greek	Lady of flowers	
Antonia	Latin, Greek	Priceless, flourishing, flower	Antoine, Antoinette, Antoinetta, Antonella, Antonellina, Tonia, Tonya, Toinette, Toni, Tony
Aphrodite	Greek	Goddess of Love	Afrodite, Aphrodesia
Apolline	Greek	Sunshine, warmth and strength	
Aretha	Greek	The best, nymph	
Aretina	Greek	Virtous	
Ariadne	Greek, Latin	Melody, very holy one	Ariana, Arianne, Arianna, Ariyaunna, Aria, Ari, Rianna
Aricia	Greek	Princess of the royal blood of Athens	
Artemisia	Greek	Belonging to Artemis	
Asia	Greek	East	
Aspasia	Greek	Welcomed	
Astra	Greek	Like a star	
Astrid	Greek, Old Norse	Star, super strength, divine strength	Astera, Astred, Asta, Astyr
Athena	Greek	Goddess of wisdom	Athene, Atena
Aure	Greek	Breeze, soft-air	

Axelia	Greek	Protector of mankind	Alexa, Alexandra, Alexis, Alexandria, Alexandrina, Alesandra, Alessandra, Allesandra, Aleksey, Alexine, Aleka, Alya, Aliki, Alejanda, Lexy, Lexie, Sandra, Zandra, Sanie, Sandy, Elke, Alexis, Alexina, Ally, Alley
Barbara	Greek, Latin	Foreign, strange, exotic, mysterious	Barbra, Bararella, Barbie, Barby, Barbs, Barb, Babette, Babs, Bobbie, Bärbel
Basha	Hebrew, Greek, Polish	Daughter of God, stranger	
Bellanca	Greek	Stronghold	
Bernice	Greek	Bringer of victory	Berry, Bunny
Calandra	Greek	Lark	Callie, Cally, Cal
Calantha	Greek	Beautiful blossoms	
Calista	Greek	Most beautiful	Cal, Kalista, Kal
Callia	Greek	Beautiful	Call, Callie, Callee
Callidora	Greek	Gift of beauty	
Calliope	Greek	Beautiful voice	
Calypso	Greek	Concealor	

Canace	Greek	Child of the wind	
Candace	Greek	White-hot, glowing, glittering	Candice, Candys, Candy, Candie, Candi, Kandy, Kan, Candis, Kandis, Kandice
Cassandra	Greek	Prophet of doom	Cassie, Cass, Cassie, Sandra, Sandy
Cassia	Greek	Champion	
Casta	Greek	Purity	
Castalia	Greek	Wife of king Delphus	
Catherine	Greek	Pure	Cathryne, Kathryn, Katherine, Katharine, Cathy, Kathie, Catie, Cadie, Caddie, Katie, Kate, Katryn, Katrina, Catrina, Trina, Cathleen, Kitty, Cate, Cat, Kat, Ky, Catriana, Catalin, Caterina, Catriona, Catlina, Cayla, Ekaterina
Celandia	Greek	The swallow	
Charis	Greek	Charity	

Charisma	Greek	Grace	Carrie, Carry
Charissa	Greek	Grace	
Charmian	Greek	A little joy	
Cherise	Greek	Grace	
Chloe	Greek	Blooming	Cloe
Christina	Greek	Annointed, follows Christ	Christine, Kristen, Kristin, Kristine, Kirsten, Kristina, Chris, Christie, Kris, Kristi, Krissie, Christiana, Christa, Chrissy, Christeena, Kristeena, Krissy, Kristy
Chruse	Greek	Golden, the Golden one	
Circe	Greek	Witch-goddess, seductive	
Claire	Latin, Greek	Bright, shining, clear	Clare, Clara, Clarice, Clarissa, Claris, Clarisse, Clarrie, Chiara, Clareta, Clarette, Claretta, Claral, Clairese
Cliantha	Greek	Flower of glory	
Clio	Greek	Praise, Muse of history	Clea, Cleo, Cleon, Cleopatra
Colette	Greek	Victory of the people	Nicolette

Cora	Greek	Maiden	Coretta, Corita, Corin, Corina, Coralee, Coralie, Corinna, Corene, Corinne, Corissa, Corisse, Cori
Cressida	Greek	Gold	
Cynara	Greek	Thistle	
Cynthia	Greek	Moon, Greek god	Cindie, Cyndi, Cindy, Cinta, Cintia, Cinzia
Cyrene	Greek	Name of a mythological nymph	
Cyrilla	Greek	Lordly, proud	
Damalis	Greek	One who gentles	
Damara	Greek	Gentle girl	
Damaris	Greek, Hebrew	Heifer	Maris
Daphne	Greek	Laurel, bay tree, victory	Daphnis
Dasha	Greek	Gift of God	
Deianira	Greek	Wife of Heracles	
Delbin	Greek	Dolphin, flower name	
Delia	Greek	Visible from Delos	Bedelia
Delphine	Greek	Calmness	
Denise	Greek	Of Dionysus	Deniece, Deniese, Denice, Denyse, Denyce, Deneise, Dennice
Desdemona	Greek	Ill-fated one, misery	
Dianthe	Greek	Divine flower	
Dionne	Greek	Divine queen	Dion, Dione
Dora	Greek	Gift	Dore, Dori
Doria	Greek	Place name	

Dorinda	Greek	Gift of God, beautiful one	
Doris	Greek	A Dorian woman, of the sea	Dorris, Dorice, Dore, Dory, Dori
Dorota	Greek, Spanish	God's gift	
Dorothy	Greek	A gift of God	Dorothea, Dottie, Dot, Dotson, Dolly, Dolley, Dotty
Dreama	Greek	Joyous music	
Dyna	Greek	Powerful	Dynean
Dysis	Greek	Sunset	
Ebony	English/Greek	Dark beauty, a hard wood	Ebonie, Ebonee
Echo	Greek	A nymph, repeated voice	
Efterpi	Greek	Pretty in face	Effie, Teppi
Eirene	Greek	Peace	
Eleanor	Greek	Light, mercy	Elie, Ella, Ellie, Elliana, Eleanore, Eleanora, Elinor, Elinore, Nell, Leonore, Leonora, Eliana
Electra	Greek	Bright, the shining one	
Eleni	Greek	Light or torch	
Elina	Greek, Hindu	Pure, intelligent	
Elissa	Greek	Queen of Carthage	
Elodie	Greek	Marshy, white blossom	
Eranthe	Greek	Spring flower	
Erasma	Greek	Amiable	
Erianthe	Greek	Sweet as many flowers	
Eudocia	Greek	Esteemed	
Eulalia	Greek	Fair of speech	
Eunice	Greek	Victorious	Eunyce, Unice
Euphrosyne	Greek	Joy	
Evadine	Greek	From Greek mythology	

Evadne	Greek	A water-nymph	
Evangelia	Greek	One who brings good news	
Evangeline	Greek	Like an angel	Evangelyn, Evangaline, Evangalyne
Evanthe	Greek	Flower	
Gaea	Greek	Goddess of the Earth	Gaia
Galatea	Greek	Milk-white	
Gelasia	Greek	Predisposed to laughter	
Georgia	Greek	Farmer, to work the earth	Georgea, Georgina, Georgianna, Georgine, Georgette, Georgeen, Georgeena, Georgeanne, Georgienne, Giorgia, Georgie, Georgy, Gina, Gerda, Gruzia, Jirka, Jirca, Jirina, Jorgina
Graeae	Greek	Gray ones	
Haidee	Greek	Modest	
Hali	Greek, Hebrew	Sea; necklace, place name	
Hallie	Greek	Thinking of the sea	
Helen	Greek	Bright one, torchlight	Helena, Helaine, Helene, Elin
Hesper	Greek	Evening star	
Hyacinth	Greek	Hyacinth flower	
Hypatia	Greek	Highest	
Ianthe	Greek	Violet-colored flower	
Idola	Greek	Idolized	
Iona	Greek	Flower name, purple jewel	
Irene	Greek	Peace	
Iris	Greek	Rainbow, a play of colours	Iria
Isadora	Greek	Gift of the moon	

Isaura	Greek	Soft air	
Ivy	Greek	Ivy plant, a wine	Ivie
Jacinda	Greek	Beautiful	
Jacinthe	Greek	Hyacinth	
Jeno	Greek	Heaven, well-born	
Kaethe	Greek	Pure	
Kaia	Greek	Earth	
Kairos	Greek	Goddess from Jupiter	
Kalika	Greek	Rosebud	Kalyca
Kalonice	Greek	Beauty's victory	
Kara	Greek	Pure	Karan, Karen, Karyn, Kasia, Katja, Kasen, Kassia, Katoka, Katrien, Kaysa
Karissa	Greek	Love, grace	Carissa, Krissy, Sissa
Katherine	Greek	Pure	Katarina, Kate, Kathryn, Kathreen, Katrin, Kathy, Katie, Kate, Katina, Katrina, Karen, Karin, Karyn, Karan, Karon, Kari, Karrie, Karry, Kara, Karina, Caren, Carin, Caryn, Cari, Carrie, Carry, Cara
Kineta	Greek	Active one	
Kirsten	Greek, Old English	Christian; stone church	Kristine, Kristi, Kirstin, Kirstie, Kirsty,

			Kirsti, Kiersten, Kier
Kolina	Greek	Pure	
Koren	Greek	Maiden	Kori, Korry, Korrie
Kynthia	Greek	Born under the sign of Cancer	
Laria	Greek	The stars are mine	
Larissa	Greek, Russian	Name of a city, mythical woman; cheerful one	
Layna	Greek	Light, truth	Laynie
Leah	Hebrew, Greek, Assyrian	Cow, weary one; glad tidings; mistress, ruler	Lea, Lia, Liah, Lee, Leatrice
Leandra	Greek	Lion woman	
Lena	Latin, Greek	Alluring, temptress; light	Lina, Lenore, Leonore, Leonora, Leonne
Letha	Greek	Forgetful, oblivion	Lethia, Leitha, Leithia, Leda, Leta
Litsa	Greek	One who brings good news	
Livana	Greek	Goddess	Livanna, Livania, Livanya
Lotus	Greek	Dreamlike, lotus flower	
Lydia	Greek	Woman from Persia, beauty	Lydie, Lidia
Lyris	Greek	Player of the lyre	
Macaria	Greek	Daughter of Hercules and Deianara	
Maeve	Greek, Latin	Goddess; a purple flower	
Maia	Greek, Latin	Nurse, mother, goddess of spring; great	
Mariam	Greek	Wife of Herod	Mariamne
Marigold	Greek	A flower	Mari,

			Golda, Goldie
Marilee	Greek	Bitterness	Marlee, Mery-Lee
Marmara	Greek	Radiant	
Medea	Greek, Latin	Ruling; middle child	Medora, Media, Madora
Megan	Greek, Gaelic, Welsh	Mighty, strong able, pearl	Meggy, Meghan, Meagan, Megann, Meggy, Meggie, Meg, Megs, Megless
Megara	Greek	Wife of Hercules	
Mclanctha	Greek	Black flower	Melantha
Melanie	Greek	Dressed in black, dark	Melany, Melane, Melani, Melania, Melloney, Melonie, Melony, Milena, Melanya, Mellie, Melly, Mel, Mela
Melba	Greek, Latin	Slender, soft; mallow flower	Melva, Malva
Melia	Greek	Nymph daugher of Oceanus	
Melinda	Greek	Gentle one	Malinda, Malina, Malinde, Malena, Melina, Minda, Mindy, Mallie, Mally, Linda,

			Lindy
Melissa	Greek	Bee, honey	Melicent, Mellissa, Millicent, Melisent, Melita, Melisse, Meli, Mellie, Melly, Mel, Millie, Milly, Missy, Lisa, Lissa, Lis
Melody	Greek	Song	Melodie, Melly, Mellie
Minerva	Greek, Latin	Power; thinker	Minette, Minnie, Minny
Minta	Greek	Mint	Mintha, Araminta, Mint
Mona	Latin, Greek, Gaelic, Italian	Peaceful; individual; noble one; My lady	
Muriel	Greek, Irish, Latin	Myrrh; sea-bright; angel of June	Murial, Meriel, Muireall
Myrtle	Greek	A flower, symbol of victory	Myrta, Myrtia, Myrtis, Mirtle, Mertle, Mertice, Mert, Myrtice, Myrtilla

Naia	Greek	Flowing	
Naida	Greek	Water nymph	Naiad, Naia, Naiia, Nayad, Nyad
Narcissa	Greek	Self-love	Narcisse
Narella	Greek	Bright one	Narelle, Relly, Relle, Rell
Nellie	Greek	The bright one	Nelly, Nellis, Nelle, Nell, Nela, Nelda, Nelia, Nella, Nelita, Nelina, Nellwyn
Neola	Greek	Youthful	
Neoma	Greek	New moon	Neona
Nerin	Greek	A Nereid, one from the sea	
Neysa	Greek	Pure	
Nicia	Greek	Victorious army	Nicanor
Nicole	Greek	Victorious people	Nichole, Nicola, Nikki, Nika, Nickie, Nicky, Nichola, Nicci, Nichelle, Nikolia, Nicoline, Nicolette, Nikole, Colette, Collette, Cosette, Lacole, Nykole, Nyky, Nykky, Nykki, Nyki
Niobe	Greek	Fern	

Nora	Greek, Latin	The bright one; honor, light	Norah, Norine, Noreen, Norina
Nyx	Greek	Night	
Obelia	Greek	Pillar of strength	
Odessa	Greek	Odyssey, journey, voyage	
Olympia	Greek	of Mount Olympus, heavenly	Olympe, Olimpie
Omega	Greek	Great	
Ophelia	Greek	Useful, wise	Ofelia, Ofilia, Ophelie, Phelia
Ophira	Greek	Gold	Oprah
Oriana	Latin, Greek	Dawn; east	Oralia, Orelle, Orlanna, Oria
Pamela	Greek	Honeyed	Pamyla, Pamilla, Pamella, Pamelia, Pamelyn, Pamelina, Pammy, Pammie, Pam
Pandora	Greek	Talented one	Pan, Dora, Dory, Dorothy, Theodore, Theodora, Endora, Dorothea
Pegeen	Greek	A pearl	
Pelagia	Greek	From the sea	Pelga, Pelgia, Pelagie
Penelope	Greek	Weaver	Penny, Penney, Pen
Penthea	Greek	Fifth, mourner	
Peony	Greek	Flower name	

Persephone	Greek	Goddess of the underworld	Persa, Perse, Percy, Fanny
Phedra	Greek	Shining one	Phaidra, Phaedra, Phae
Philadelphia	Greek	Brotherly love	
Philana	Greek	Adoring	Philene, Philina, Philida, Philantha, Philander, Falana
Philippa	Greek	Horse lover	Philippine, Felipe, Felipa, Philly, Philia,
Philomena	Greek	Song lover, friend, lover of the moon	Filomena, Philomen
Phineas	Greek, Egyptian	Oracle; dark-skinned	Phinny, Phin, Finn, Pincus, Pinchas, Pinchos
Phoena	Greek	Mystical bird, purple	
Phyllis	Greek	Leafy branch, dear	Phillis, Phylys, Philicia, Philida, Filida, Philly, Phil, Phyl
Psyche	Greek	The soul	
Pyrena	Greek	Fiery	
Pythia	Greek	Prophet	
Raissa	Old French, Greek	Thinker; rose	Raisa
Rena	Greek, Hebrew	Peace; joyous song	
Rhea	Greek, Latin	Stream, mother; poppy	Ria, Rea
Rhoda	Greek	Rose	Rhodia, Rhodie, Rodie, Roe
Rhodanthe	Greek	Flower of the rose bush	
Rita	Greek	Pearl, precious	
Rizpah	Greek	Hope	Ritzpa
Rose	Latin, Greek	A flower	Rosa, Rosie,

			Rosey, Roz, Rozsi, Rosalie, Rosalee, Rosalia, Rosetta, Rosette, Rosina, Rosena, Rasia, Rois, Rosita, Rosebud, Rosabell, Rosly, Roslin, Rosamund, Rosmund, Rosemonde, Rozamund, Roanee, Roanna, Rosaleen, Rosellen, Roselle, Rosella, Rosemary, Rosemarie,
Rue	Latin, Greek	A herb name; regret	
Saba	Greek	Woman of Sheba	
Sandrine	Greek	Helper and defender of mankind	Sandra
Sapphira	Greek	Blue jewel	Saphira, Sapphire
Seema	Greek, Hindu	Symbol	
Selena	Greek	Moon	Selina, Selene, Selinda, Selly, Sellie, Sela, Selia, Sena, Celena, Celina, Celene, Celie, Celia

Sibley	Greek	Prophetess	Sibyl, Sibylle, Sybil, Sybyl, Sybille, Sibille, Sibeal, Sybilline, Sibby, Sibbi, Sib, Cybil, Cybill
Sirena	Greek	Siren	
Sophie	Greek	Wisdom	Sofi, Sophia, Sofia, Sofie, Sophy, Sophronia, Sadhbh, Zofka
Sophronia	Greek	Foresighted	
Stacia	Greek	One who shall rise again	
Stefania	Greek	Crown	Stephanie, Stephannie, Stepania, Stephania, Stefanie, Stephana, Stephanya, Steffie, Steffi, Stef, Stepha, Stefa, Fannie, Fanny, Stefka
Stella	Greek, Latin	A star	Stela, Stellar, Star, Starr, Starla, Starling
Stesha	Greek	Crowned-one	
Syna	Greek	Two together	
Tabitha	Greek, Hebrew	Gazelle, roe-buck	Tabatha, Tabbie,

			Tabbi, Tabby
Talia	Hebrew, Greek, Australian Aboriginal	Dew from heaven, blooming, near water	Talya, Tally, Tai, Talitha
Taryn	Greek	Queen	
Tekla	Greek	Divine fame	Thekla
Terentia	Greek	Guardian	
Tess	Greek	Fourth born	Tessie, Tessy
Thais	Greek	The bond	
Thalassa	Greek	From the sea	
Thalia	Greek	Blooming, plentiful	Taylie, Taylee, Thalius
Thea	Greek, Laos	Goddess, sort	
Thelma	Greek	Nursing	Telma
Theodora	Greek	Gift of God	Theora, Theda, Teodora, Theodosia, Thedora, Tedra, Feodora, Fedora, Dora, Theone, Theophania, Theophilia
Theone	Greek	Godly	
Thera	Greek	wild	
Theresa	Greek	Reaper	Teresa, Teressa, Therese, Toireasa, Teri, Terri, Terry, Tessa, Tess, Tessie, Tessy, Tracey, Tracie, Tracy, Tressa,

			Tessica
Thisbe	Greek	Where the doves live	
Thomasa	Greek	Twin	Thomasina, Thomasine, Tomasina, Tommie, Tommy, Tammy, Tamsen, Tamsin, Tamson, Thomasssa
Thyra	Greek	Shield-bearer	
Tia	Spanish, Greek	Aunt, princess	Tianna, Tiana
Tiara	Greek, Latin	Turban, flower name	Teara
Tienette	Greek	Crowned with laurel	Tiena, Tien
Timandra	Greek	Daughter of hero Tyndareus	
Timothea	Greek	Honoring God	Thea, Timora
Titania	Greek	Giant	
Titian	Greek	Red-gold	
Urania	Greek	Heavenly, muse of Astronomy	
Uriana	Greek	The unknown	
Vanessa	Greek	A butterfly	Vannia, Vanna, Vannie, Vanora, Nessa, Nessie, Nessy, Venissa

Vasiliki	Greek	Basil	
Vesna	Croatian, Greek	Goddess of spring	
Voleta	Greek	Veiled one	Velita
Xandy	Greek	Protector of man	
Xanthe	Greek	Yellow, fair hair	
Xenia	Greek	Hospitable	Xena
Xylia	Greek	Wood dweller	
Xylona	Greek	From the forest	Xylina, Zylona, Zylina
Yolanda	Greek	Violet flower, modest	Yolande, Yolantha, Iolanthe, Iolande, Eolande, Jolanda, Jolaunda, Jo, Yo, Landa
Zandra	Greek	Defender of mankind	Zandria, Andria, Andra
Zanita	Greek	Long teeth	
Zebina	Greek	One who is gifted	
Zelia	Greek	Zeal	
Zena	Greek	Alive	
Zenaide	Greek	One who has devoted her life to God	
Zenia	Greek	Hospitable	
Zenobia	Greek	Of Zeus	Zenobie, Zena, Zenna, Zenina, Zinovia
Zera	Greek	Seeds	
Zeva	Greek	Sword	
Zinaida	Greek	Of Zeus	Zenais, Zina
Zoe	Greek	Life	Zoë, Zoey, Zoé

Zora	Slavic, Greek	Golden dawn	Zorah, Zoradah, Zohra, Zarya, Zoranna, Zorina, Zoriana, Zori, Zorie, Zorry
Zosima	Greek	Lively	

Hawaiian Female Baby Names

Name	Origin	Meaning	Similiar Names
Akela	Hawaiian	Noble	
Alana	Gaelic, Hawaiian	Fair, beautiful, offering	Alaina, Alyn, Allyn, Lani, Allie, Ally, Alli, Lanny, Alun, Alanna, Laina, Lane, Laney, Elaine, Alona
Anani	Hawaiian	Orange tree	
Aolani	Hindu, Hawaiian	Cloud from Heaven	
Haimi	Hawaiian	The seeker	
Haleigha	Hawaiian	House of the rising sun	Haleah, Leigha
Iolana	Hawaiian	To soar like an eagle	
Kaili	Hawaiian	A deity	
Kalama	Hawaiian	Flaming torch	
Kalea	Hawaiian	Bright	
Keilana	Hawaiian	Adored one	
Kekona	Hawaiian	Second-born	
Kiana	Hawaiian	Moon Goddess	
Kiele	Hawaiian	Gardenia, fragrant blossom	
Lani	Hawaiian	Sky, heaven	
Lanikai	Hawaiian	Heavenly sea	
Lokelani	Hawaiian	Small red rose	
Malu	Hawaiian	Peacefulness	
Mily	Hawaiian	Beautiful	
Nalani	Hawaiian	Calmness of the skies	
Noelani	Hawaiian	Beautiful girl from heaven	
Okelani	Hawaiian	From heaven	
Oliana	Hawaiian	Oleander	
Peni	Hawaiian	Weaver	
Roselani	Hawaiian	Heavenly rose	

Hebrew Female Baby Names

Name	Origin	Meaning	Similiar Names
Aaliyah	Arabic, Hebrew	High exalted, to ascend	Aleah, Alea, Aleaseya, Aliya, Alia, Aleeya, Aliyah, Allyiah
Abigail	Latin, Hebrew	Head of a monastery, a father's joy	Abbey, Abbe, Abbie, Abby, Abagail, Abigayle, Abigale, Gail, Abilio, Abihail
Abira	Hebrew	Strong	
Abra	Hebrew	Father of a multitude	
Achazia	Hebrew	The Lord holds	
Ada	Teutonic, Hebrew	Happy, ornament	Adah
Adalia	Hebrew, Arabic, German	Refuge of God, just, noble one	
Adamina	Hebrew	Daughter of the Earth	
Adelaide	Hebrew, Latin	Noble kind, adorned	Adalia, Adeline, Aline, Adele, Ellie, Addie, Elle, Adelle, Della, Adailia, Adalee, Adara, Adah, Eda, Etta, Ady, Adela, Adalheld
Adena	Hebrew	Delicate, sensual	Adina, Adinna, Adenna
Aderes	Hebrew	One who protects	
Adie	Hebrew	Ornament	
Adina	Hebrew	Beautiful, Adorned, Slender	
Ahava	Hebrew	Name of a river, love	
Ailsa	Hebrew	Consecrated to God	
Akiva	Hebrew	Protect	
Aliza	Hebrew	Joyous	
Alumit	Hebrew	Secret	
Amissa	Hebrew	Friend	

Anke	Hebrew	Grace	Anka
Anne	Hebrew	Gracious	Ann, Anna, Annis, Annys, Anya, Anja, Anika, Annika, Annie, Annice, Anita, Anca, Anneka, Annette, Ana, Anita, Annette, Nanette, Anitia, Anushka, Anuschka
Araminta	Hebrew	Lofty	
Arashel	Hebrew	Strong and protected hill	
Arella	Hebrew	Angel messenger	
Ariel	Hebrew	Lioness of God	Arial, Aryel, Ario, Ari, Ariella, Ariela, Ariele, Arielle, Alli, Rel
Asa	Hebrew	Healer	
Asenka	Hebrew	Graceful	
Asisa	Hebrew	Ripe	
Astera	Hebrew	Flower name	
Atara	Hebrew	A crown	
Athalia	Hindu, Hebrew	God is exalted, the Lord is mighty	
Aviva	Hebrew	Springtime	Avital, Avi, Avia, Avivah
Ayala	Hebrew	Gazelle, goat	
Ayla	Hebrew	Oak tree	
Azalia	Hebrew	Spared by jehovah	Azaria
Bara	Hebrew	To choose	
Basha	Hebrew, Greek, Polish	Daughter of God, stranger	
Bathsheba	Hebrew	Daughter of the oath	Batsheva, Bathshua, Batya, Basia, Basya, Sheba
Beth	Hebrew	House of god	Elizabeth, Betty
Bethany	Hebrew	House	Bethanie, Betheny, Bethesda, Bethel, Beth, Annie, Bethannie
Bina	Hindu, Hebrew	A musical instrument, intelligence	

Bracha	Hebrew	A blessing	
Buffy	Hebrew	God's promise	
Carmen	Hebrew, Latin	Garden, field of fruit, song	Carmel, Karmen, Karmel, Carmelita, Karmelita, Carmelle, Karmelle, Carmine, Carmita
Chanah	Hebrew	Grace	
Chaya	Hebrew	Life	
Daba	Hebrew	Kind words, bee swarm	
Dalia	Hebrew	A branch, to draw water	Dahlia
Damaris	Greek, Hebrew	Heifer	Maris
Daniela	Hebrew	My judge is the Lord	Dania, Danett, Dannett, Danet, Danielle, Danelle, Nellc, Nelly, Dana, Danae, Danna, Daniella, Danice, Danya, Danita, Dada
Dara	Hebrew, Persian	Compassion, wisdom, Angel of rains and rivers	
Davan	Hebrew	Beloved one	Davida
Davine	Hebrew	The loved	Davina, Davita
Daya	Hebrew	Bird	
Dayla	Hebrew	To draw water, branch or bough	
Deborah	Hebrew	A bee, to speak kind words	Debra, Debrah, Debbie, Debby, Deb, Debo, Devora, Devorah
Delilah	Hebrew	Delicate, amorous	Delila, Lila, Lilah
Dena	Hebrew, Native American	Vindicated, valley	Denna
Dinah	Hebrew	Vindicated, judgement	Dina, Deena, Deanna
Edna	Hebrew	Pleasure, delight	
Edria	Hebrew	Mighty	
Efrosini	Hebrew	A fawn or a bird	

Eilis	Hebrew, Celtic	God's oath	
Eleora	Hebrew	The Lord is my light	
Elisabeth	Hebrew/Germanic	God's oath	Elizabeth, Ellyzabeth, Elise, Elyse, Elysia, Eliza, Beth, Bess, Liz, Lizzy, Elsa, Elsie, Elpeth, Elsbeth, Lisbeth, Lizzie, Liza, Ellie, Bess, Betty, Bette, Bettie, Betsy, Aliza, Arlise, Arlisa, Libby, Isabel, Isabelle, Isabella, Ilse
Elisha	Hebrew	Jehovah is God	Elisheba
Ellen	Hebrew	Light, mercy	Ellyn, Elen, Elyn, Ellin, Elin, Elena
Else	Hebrew	Consecrated to God	
Emanuela	Hebrew	God is with us	Emmanuella, Manuella
Endora	Hebrew	Fountain	
Erzsebet	Hebrew	Devoted to God	
Eva	Hebrew	Life	Evacsa, Ewa, Eve, Evette, Evie, Evita, Evonne, Evy, Ev, Ava
Evelina	Hebrew	Life-giving	
Gabrielle	Hebrew	God is my strength	Gabby, Gabriela, Gabbryela, Gabi, Gabriella, Gaby, Gavrila, Gavra, Galia, Galya, Gabi
Gali	Hebrew	Spring, fountain	
Galya	Hebrew	God is redeemed	
Gana	Hebrew	Garden	
Geva	Hebrew	Hill	
Gilana	Hebrew	Joy	
Hadara	Hebrew	Bedecked in beauty	
Hadassa	Hebrew	Flowering myrtle	Hadasa, Hadaseh
Hali	Greek, Hebrew	Sea; necklace, place name	
Hana	Japanese, Hebrew	Flower, blossom; graceful, merciful	

Hannah	Hebrew	Grace of God	Hana, Hanna
Hanne	Hebrew	Gracious	
Hava	Hebrew	Life	
Heba	Hebrew	Gift from God	
Hedia	Hebrew	Voice of the Lord	Hedya
Hedva	Hebrew	Joy	
Ideh	Hebrew	Praise	
Ilana	Hebrew	Sunshine	Iyana, Lana, Ana, Ilani
Iva	Hebrew, Japanese	God's great gift, yew tree	
Ivana	Hebrew	God is gracious	
Jacqueline	Hebrew	Supplanter	Jamie, Jacobienne, Jaclyn, Jackie, Jaclyn, Jacky, Jacki
Jada	Hebrew	Wise	
Jael	Hebrew	To ascend	
Jaen	Hebrew	Ostrich	
Jamee	Hebrew	Supplanter, one who replaces	Jamie, Jaimee, Jaimy, Jayme, Jamie, Jaymie, Jay
Jane	Hebrew	Gracious, merciful, God is gracious	Shana, Sheena, Shona, Sian, Jana, Jean, Jeanette, Jeanne, Jeannie, Jeanie, Jeanise, Jeanita, Janice, Janine, Janet, Janae, Jan, Gianna
Janna	Hebrew	Flourishing	
Jardena	Hebrew	To flow downward	
Jensine	Hebrew	God is gracious	Jensyn, Jensi, Jeni
Jessica	Hebrew	God's grace	Jessicka, Jessykah, Jess, Jesse, Jessy, Jessie
Jezebel	Hebrew	Follower of idols	
Joakima	Hebrew	The Lord will judge	Joan, Joannie, Joann
Joanne	Hebrew	God is gracious	Joan, Joann, Joanna, Johanna, Giovanna, Juanita, Juaniqua, Johanne, Joas, Jurnel, Joetta,

			Shawna
Jobey	Hebrew	Persecuted	
Jobina	Hebrew	The persecuted	
Joelle	Hebrew	The Lord is willing	
Joelliane	Hebrew	Jehova is God	
Jonina	Hebrew	Dove	Jonna
Jora	Hebrew	Autumn rain	
Jordane	Hebrew	Descendant, flowing down	Jordana, Jori, Jordyn, Jordene, Jordann
Josephine	Hebrew	God will increase	Josefina, Josephina, Giuseppina, Jody, Josie
Judith	Hebrew	Praise, admired	Jude, Judit, Judy
Justine	Hebrew, Latin	Just, true	Justina, Giustina
Kadisha	Hebrew	Holy	Kadischa, Kadiza
Kalanit	Hebrew	Flower name	
Kayla	Hebrew	Crown of laurels	Kaila, Kaylynn, Kailyn, Kaylene, Kaylah, Kayln, Kay
Kazia	Hebrew	Plant with cinnamon-like bark	
Kefira	Hebrew	Young lioness	
Keturah	Hebrew	Fragrance	
Ketzia	Hebrew	Surface, cinnamon-like bark	
Kezia	Hebrew	Cassia, cinnamon	Keesha, Keziah, Ketzia, Kezzy, Keisha, Keishia, Keshia, Lakeisha
Lailie	Hebrew	Born during light	
Leah	Hebrew, Greek, Assyrian	Cow, weary one; glad tidings; mistress, ruler	Lea, Lia, Liah, Lee, Leatrice
Ledah	Hebrew	Birth	
Lexine	Hebrew	Helper and defender of mankind	
Lia	Hebrew	Dependence	

Lilith	Sumerian, Assyrian, Hebrew	Ghost; storm goddess; spirit of the night	Lilyth, Lily
Lisa	Hebrew	Consecrated to God	Lisette, Lisetta, Liza
Madeline	Hebrew	Woman from Magdala, one who is elevated, a high tower	Marlene, Magdalene, Magdalen, Magdalena, Maigarena, Mayalen, Madeleine, Madleen, Madalynn, Madelynne, Madelaine, Madalena, Madelon, Madelyn, Madlin, Madigan, Marleen, Marlena, Marline, Maighdlin, Maudlin, Malina, Magda, Mady, Maddy, Maddie, Matty, Mala, Mae, May, Lena, Lene, Madeline,Magdaline, Maddalena
Magda	Hebrew	High tower, one who is elevated	
Magena	Native American, Hebrew	The coming moon; a covering, protection	
Mahala	Native American, Hebrew, Arabic	Woman; tenderness; marrow	Mahalah, Mahalar, Mahela, Mahalia, Mahelia, Mehala
Mahalia	Hebrew	Affection	
Malca	Hebrew	Queen	Malka
Malina	Hebrew, Hindu	Tower, dark	Malini
Malka	Hebrew	Queen	
Mangena	Hebrew	Melody	
Maria	Hebrew	Bitter	Mary, Marya, Mariah, Marie, Malia, Ri, Mar
Mariasha	Egyptian, Hebrew	Perfect one; bitter, with sorrow	
Maridel	Hebrew	Bitter	Meridel

Mariel	Hebrew	Bitter	Marielle, Mariella, Marietta, Mariette, Marette, Maretta
Marilyn	Hebrew	Bitter	Mary-Lynn, Maralin, Marilin, Marylin, Marlyn, Marlin, Marly, Mari, Lynn
Marna	Hebrew	Rejoice	Marnie, Marni, Marny, Marnette, Marne
Marnina	Hebrew	Cause of joy	
Mary	Hebrew	Bitter	Mari, Merry, Marie, Maria, Miriam, Marian, Mame, Mamie, Maymie, Mayme, May, Mally, Molly, Polly, Mara, Maretta, Marel, Marella, Maren, Marlo, Mariette, Marieta, Meriel, Mimi, Minette, Minnie, Minny, Mitzi, Madonna, Marilla, Marla, Marya, Muriel, Manon, Manette, Marija, Marika, Maire, Mare, Marquita, Maure, Mairin, Mair, Maura, Maureen, Moira, Moire, Moya, Muire, Masha, Mairi, Mariya, Mashia, Mash, Mariath
Mathea	Hebrew	Gift of God	Matthea, Mathia, Mattea, Mathia
May	Hebrew	Bitter	Mae, Mai, Maia, Maya, Maye, Mayes, Mays, Maize
Meira	Hebrew	Light	

Michaela	Hebrew	Like God	Michaelina, Michaeline, Michelina, Micaela, Mikaela, Miguela, Michelle, Nichelle, Shelly, Shell, Michal, Micheline, Michelyn, Mickey, Mikhaeli, Mikaeli
Minna	Old German, Scottish, Hebrew	Love; mother; bitterness	Mina, Minette, Minetta, Minda, Myna, Mindy
Mira	Latin, Spanish; Hebrew	Wonder; aim; light of God	Myra, Mirila, Mirella, Mirelle, Mirielle, Myrilla
Miriam	Hebrew	Bitter	Miryam, Myriam, Mimi, Mitzi, Miri, Mims, Mimsie, Meryem, Mirjam, Mirem
Moria	Hebrew	My teacher is God	Moriah, Moriel, Morit, Moryah
Moselle	Hebrew	Taken from water	Mozelle, Mosheh
Nancy	Hebrew	Full of grace	Nancee, Nansey, Nansee, Nana, Nanny, Nan, Nanette, Nannette, Nanine, Nanice, Nance
Nanna	Hebrew	Graceful one	
Naomi	Hebrew, Japanese	Pleasent one; above all, beauty	Naoma, Noami, Mimi, Mimsy, Mims, Nomi, Omie
Nataniella	Hebrew	Gift of God	Natanielle, Nathania, Natania, Nathanielle
Naysa	Hebrew	Miracle of God	
Nediva	Hebrew	Noble and generous	
Neria	Hebrew	Lamp of God, angel	
Netta	Hebrew	A plant or shrub	

Nina	Spanish, Hebrew	Girl; grace	Ninya, Ninette, Ninon
Nira	Hebrew	Of the loom	
Nitzana	Hebrew	Blossom	
Odelia	Old German; Hebrew	Little wealthy one; praise God	Odella, Odelinda, Odilia, Odelette
Odera	Hebrew	Plough	
Oralia	Latin, Hebrew	Golden; light	Orel, Orelda, Oriole, Orlene, Orlena, Orpah, Oralee, Oralie, Oral, Ora, Orah, Oria, Orlie, Orly, Orabel
Pazia	Hebrew	golden	
Penina	Hebrew	Jewel, coral	Peninah, Peninna, Peninit, Penny, Peni, Nina
Rachel	Hebrew	Little lamb, an ewe, one with purity	Rachael, Raychel, Rachele, Rah'zell, Rahel, Raquel, Ray, Shelley, Shelly, Shellie, Chelle, Chellie
Raizel	Hebrew	Rose	Rayzel, Razel
Raphaella	Hebrew	Healed by God	Rafaella
Rayna	Hebrew	pure, clean	
Rebecca	Hebrew	Bound, tied	Rebekah, Rebeckah, Rebeccah, Rebeca, Rebeka, Rebeque, Rebekka, Rebakah, Rebequa, Becky, Bekki, Becca, Becha, Becka, Riba, Reba, Riva, Reeba, Ree, Rivka, Rifka, Rivca, Rivy
Rena	Greek, Hebrew	Peace; joyous song	
Rishona	Hebrew	First	
Ruth	Hebrew	Compassionate friend	Ruthie, Ruthanne

Sabra	Arabic, Hebrew	Thorny cactus; to rest	
Saloma	Hebrew	Peace	Salome
Samara	Hebrew, Latin	Mountain, outlook, ruled by God, guarded by God; seedling	
Samuela	Hebrew	Her name is God	Samuella, Samella
Sarah	Hebrew	Princess	Sara, Sari, Sarri, Sary, Sarrie, Sarene, Sarina, Sarine, Sarita, Sairne, Sarett, Sadie, Sadey, Zarah, Zara, Zaria
Sarai	Hebrew	Quarrelsome	
Sarea	Hebrew	Name of an angel	
Sela	Hebrew	A rock	
Seraphina	Hebrew	Afire, angel, seraph	Serafina, Sarafina, Serafine, Seraphine, Seraphim, Sera
Shaine	Hebrew	Beautiful	Shaina, Shaynah, Shanie, Shayna, Shay, Shanna, Shana
Shalom	Hebrew	Peace	
Sharon	Hebrew	Princess	Shari, Sharee, Shara, Sharen, Sharyn, Sharron, Charon, Sharry, Sherry, Sherri
Shawn	Hebrew	God is gracious	Shaunna, Shaun
Sheba	Hebrew	From Sheba	
Shelah	Hebrew	Request	
Shira	Hebrew	Song	Shirah, Shiri
Shobi	Hebrew	Glorious	
Shoshannah	Hebrew	Rose	Shoshanna, Shoshana, Shoshanah, Shosha
Simone	Hebrew	One who hears	Simona

Susan	Hebrew	Lily	Susannah, Susanne, Susanna, Susi, Suse, Suisan, Suzanne, Suzanna, Sosana, Susette, Suzette, Sue Anne, Sue Ellen, Susy, Susie, Soos, Suzy, Suzie, Soozie, Sue, Sukie, Sukey, Zsa Zsa
Sydelle	Hebrew	Princess	
Tabitha	Greek, Hebrew	Gazelle, roe-buck	Tabatha, Tabbie, Tabbi, Tabby
Talia	Hebrew, Greek, Australian Aboriginal	Dew from heaven, blooming, near water	Talya, Tally, Tai, Talitha
Tamara	Hebrew, Sanskrit	Palm tree, spice	Tamarah, Tamar, Tamarind, Tamika, Tamary
Tammy	Hebrew	Perfect one	Tammie
Tapanga	African, Hebrew	Sweet, unpredictable	Tata, Pangi
Tema	Hebrew	Righteous, a palm tree	
Temina	Hebrew	Honest	
Thirza	Hebrew	Sweet-natured, cypress tree	Thyrza, Tirza, Tyrza
Tivona	Hebrew	Lover of nature	
Tove	Hebrew	Good	
Uma	Hebrew, Hindu, Japanese	Nation, mother, horse	
Varda	Hebrew	Rose	
Yachne	Hebrew	Gracious	
Ydel	Hebrew	Praise	Yidel
Yesmina	Hebrew	Right hand, strength	
Yoninah	Hebrew	Dove	Yonina
Yovela	Hebrew	Rejoicing	
Zakia	Hebrew	Bright, pure	
Zambda	Hebrew	Meditation	
Zara	Hebrew, Arabic	Dawn, princess	Zarah, Zarry, Zari, Zerlinda
Zaza	Hebrew, Arabic	Movement, flowery	
Zehava	Hebrew	Golden	
Zerlinda	Hebrew	Beautiful dawn	

Zevida	Hebrew	Gift	
Zia	Hebrew, Latin	To tremble, a kind of grain	
Zila	Hebrew	Shadow	
Ziona	Hebrew	A sign	
Zisel	Hebrew	Sweet	Zysel
Zita	Hebrew, Persian	The seeker; virgin	
Zuriel	Hebrew	God is my rock	

Hindu Female Baby Names

Name	Origin	Meaning	Similiar Names
Athalia	Hindu, Hebrew	God is exalted, The Lord is mighty	
Atmaja	Hindu	Daughter	
Avanti	Hindu	Ancient Malwa	
Avasa	Hindu	Independent	
Ayushmati	Hindu	Person who has a long life	
Baka	Hindu	Crane	
Bansari	Hindu	Bansuri	
Bel	Hindu	Sacred wood apple tree	
Bhoomi	Hindu	Earth	Bhumi
Bina	Hindu, Hebrew	A musical instrument, intelligence	
Chaitra	Hindu	Aries sign	
Chhaya	Hindu	Shadow	
Chitra	Hindu	Portrait	
Damini	Hindu	Lightning	
Deepika	Hindu	A little light	
Devaki	Hindu	Black, mother of Krishna	
Devi	Hindu	Resides in heaven	
Divya	Hindu	Heavenly, brilliant	Divia
Drisana	Hindu	Daughter of the sun	
Dristi	Hindu	Sight, a form of the Devi	
Elina	Greek, Hindu	Pure, intelligent	
Gajendra	Hindu	Elephant king	
Ganesa	Hindu	Good luck	
Gauri	Hindu	Yellow	
Gayatri	Hindu	Mother of the Vedas	
Hema	Hindu	Snow, himalayas	
Hinda	Hindu	Female deer	
Inayat	Hindu	Kindness	
Indira	Hindu	India	
Indrina	Hindu	Deep	
Ishana	Hindu	Rich	
Jaina	Hindu	Good character	

Jaya	Hindu	Name of a God, victory	
Jayani	Hindu	A sakti of Ganesha	
Jayne	Hindu	Victorious	
Jyoti	Hindu	Light	
Kajal	Hindu	Eyeliner	
Kala	Hindu	Time, black	
Kamakshi	Hindu	A Devi, same as Lalita	
Kamala	Hindu	Lotus	
Kamna	Hindu	Desire	
Kanchana	Hindu	A celestial Apsara, gold	
Kantha	Hindu	Name of a God	
Karka	Hindu	Crab	
Kaveri	Hindu	Sacred river of India	
Kavindra	Hindu	Mighty poet	
Kavita	Hindu	Poem	
Kerani	Hindu	Sacred bells	
Kimatra	Hindu	Seduce	Kim
Kiran	Hindu	Ray	Kiranpal
Kirti	Hindu	Fame	
Kirti	Hindu	Fame, a form of the Devi	
Kriti	Hindu	A work of art	
Kshama	Hindu	Forgiveness, patience, a form of the Devi	
Lalasa	Hindu	Love	
Lavani	Hindu	Grace	Laboni
Lolaksi	Hindu	A sakti of Ganesha	
Madhu	Hindu	Honey	
Madhur	Hindu	Sweet	
Maitryi	Hindu	Friendship	Maitri
Mala	Hindu	Necklace	
Malati	Hindu	Small fragrant flower	Malti
Maliha	Hindu	Strong, beautiful	Mali, Malha, Hala
Malina	Hebrew, Hindu	Ttower, dark	Malini
Mamta	Hindu	Mother's love for child, wife of sage Asija	
Manda	Latin, Hindu	Lovable, harmony; Saturn, god of the fragrant	
Mandara	Hindu	Mythical tree	
Mandeep	Hindu	Light of heart	
Manisha	Hindu	Sharp intellect, genius,	

		sagacity	
Marisa	Hindu	Mother of Daksa	
Matangi	Hindu	A Devi	
Matrika	Hindu	Mother, name of goddess	
Maya	Hindu	Divine creative force in everything	
Medha	Hindu	Intelligence, a form of the Devi	
Meena	Hindu	Precious stone	Mina
Meghana	Hindu	Rain cloud	
Mela	Hindu	Religious gathering	
Mena	Hindu	mother of Menaka	
Menaka	Hindu	Celestial damsel	
Mesha	Hindu	Ram, born under the sign of Aries	
Mohini	Hindu	Most beautiful	
Naina	Hindu	Eyes	
Nanda	Hindu	A sakti of Ganesha	
Narmada	Hindu	Name of a river	
Neelam	Hindu	Sapphire	
Neerja	Hindu	Lotus flower	
Neha	Hindu	Rain	
Nidra	Hindu	A form of the Devi	
Niju	Hindu	Pansophist	Nij
Nilini	Hindu	Perpetuator of the Kuru race	
Nirvana	Hindu	Deep silence, ultimate bliss	Vana
Nisha	Hindu	Night	
Nitara	Hindu	Deeply rooted	
Nitya	Hindu	Goddess Parvati	
Niyati	Hindu	Fate	
Padma	Hindu	Goddess Lakshmi	
Parnika	Hindu	Auspicious Apsara	
Parnita	Hindu	Auspicious Apsara	
Parthivi	Hindu	The Goddess Sita	
Parvani	Hindu	Full moon	
Parvati	Hindu	The Goddess Sarasvati	
Parveen	Hindu	Star	
Payal	Hindu	Anklet	
Phoolan	Hindu	Flower	
Pivari	Hindu	A wife of Sukha	

Piyali	Hindu	Tree	
Pooja	Hindu	Prayer	Puja
Prabha	Hindu	Lustrous	
Prabhati	Hindu	Morning	
Pradeepta	Hindu	Glowing	
Pragati	Hindu	Progress	
Pragya	Hindu	Wisdom	
Prama	Hindu	Knowing truth	
Pramada	Hindu	Woman	
Pranati	Hindu	Prayer	
Prapti	Hindu	Gain	
Prashanti	Hindu	Peace	
Pratima	Hindu	Image	
Preeti	Hindu	Love	
Preyasi	Hindu	Beloved	
Prita	Hindu	Dear one	
Priti	Hindu	Satisfaction, renowned wife of Pulastya/Sukha	
Pritika	Hindu	Beloved	Priyal, Priyam
Priya	Hindu	Loved one, darling	Priyasha
Purvaja	Hindu	Elder sister	
Pusti	Hindu	Nourishment, a form of the Devi, wife of Ganapati	
Radhika	Hindu	A form of the Devi, 5th Sakti, wife of Krishna	
Ramya	Hindu	Elegant, beautiful	
Rani	Hindu	A queen	
Rati	Hindu	A Devi	
Rekha	Hindu	Straight line	
Reshma	Hindu	Silky	
Revati	Hindu	Wife of Balarama	
Riddhi	Hindu	Siddhi will follow	
Rina	Hindu	Queen	Reena, Riena
Rohana	Hindu	Sandalwood	
Roshni	Hindu	Light	
Rudrani	Hindu	A wife of Shiva	
Sachi	Japanese, Hindu	Bliss-child; wife of Indra	
Sagara	Hindu	Ocean	
Saheli	Hindu	Friend	Sakhi, Sakina
Sahiba	Hindu	Lady	
Sahila	Hindu	Guide	

Sajili	Hindu	Decorated	
Sajni	Hindu	Beloved	
Sakti	Hindu	Energy, goodness	
Saloni	Hindu	Dear, beautiful	
Sampriti	Hindu	Attachment	
Sanchay	Hindu	Collection	Sandhaya, Sandhya
Sandya	Hindu	Sunset time, name of a God	
Sangita	Hindu	Musical	
Sanjna	Hindu	Wife of the Sun	
Sanjula	Hindu	Beautiful	Sanjushree, Sohni
Sapna	Hindu	Dream	
Sarasvati	Hindu	A Goddess	
Sarika	Hindu	Thrush	
Sarisha	Hindu	Charming	
Sarita	Hindu	Stream, river	
Sarmistha	Hindu	A daughter of Vrsaparvan	
Saryu	Hindu	A river in Ramayana	
Satyavati	Hindu	Mother of Vyasa	
Savarna	Hindu	Daughter of the ocean	
Savita	Hindu	Sun	
Savitri	Hindu	A form of the Devi, 4th Sakti	
Seema	Greek, Hindu	Symbol	
Sesha	Hindu	Serpent who symbolizes time	
Sevati	Hindu	White rose	
Sevita	Hindu	Beloved	
Shaili	Hindu	Style	
Shamita	Hindu	Peace maker	
Shanata	Hindu	Peaceful	
Shantah	Hindu	Peace, name of a God	Shanta, Shanti
Sheetal	Hindu	Cool	
Shreya	Hindu	Auspicious	
Shri	Hindu	Lustre	
Shrijani	Hindu	Creative	
Shruti	Hindu	Hearing	
Siddhi	Hindu	Then you must have a Riddhi	
Simoni	Hindu	Obedient	
Simran	Hindu	God's Gift	

Smita	Hindu	Smiling	Susmita
Smriti	Hindu	Recollection, a form of the Devi	
Somatra	Hindu	Excelling the moon	
Sona	Hindu	Gold	
Sonakshi	Hindu	Golden eye	
Sonal	Hindu	Golden	Sonali
Sonika	Hindu	Golden	
Sraddha	Hindu	Faith, a wife of Shiva	
Subhadra	Hindu	A wife of Arjuna	
Subhaga	Hindu	A fortunate person	
Subhuja	Hindu	Auspicious Apsara	
Sudevi	Hindu	Wife of Krishna	
Sunita	Hindu	A daughter of Dharma	Sunrita
Suparna	Hindu	Leafy	
Suprabha	Hindu	Radiant	
Supriya	Hindu	Su means good and "Priya" means "loved one"	
Surabhi	Hindu	Wish-yielding cow	
Suravinda	Hindu	A beautiful Yaksa	
Surotama	Hindu	Auspicious Apsara	
Sushanti	Hindu	Peace	
Sushmita	Hindu	Smiling	Susmita
Susila	Hindu	Wife of Krishna, clever in amorous sciences	
Swarupa	Hindu	Truth	
Tara	Celtic, Gaelic, Hindu	Rocky hill, tower	Taria, Taryn
Tina	Old English, Hindu	River	Tyna
Trishna	Hindu	Thirst, a form of the Devi	
Tulasi	Hindu	A Devi	
Tusti	Hindu	Peace, happiness, a for of the Devi	
Uma	Hebrew, Hindu, Japanese	Nation, mother, horse	
Uma	Hindu	Wife of Shiva	
Unnati	Hindu	Progress	
Urmila	Hindu	Wife of Lakshmana	
Urvasi	Hindu	Most beautiful of Apsaras	
Uttara	Hindu	Mother of Pariksit	
Varsha	Hindu	Rain	
Varuni	Hindu	A goddess	
Vasanta	Hindu	Spring	
Vasavi	Hindu	Mental daughter of the Pitrs	
Vasumati	Hindu	Apsara of unequalled splendour	

Vidya	Hindu	Wisdom, knowledge	
Vimala	Hindu	Pure, sakti of the Gayatri Devi	
Vinata	Hindu	Humble, mother of Garuda	
Vinaya	Hindu	Good behaviour	
Visala	Hindu	Celestial Apsara	
Vrinda	Hindu	Virtue and strength	
Yaksha	Hindu	A sister of Daksha	

Hopi Indian Female Baby Names

Name	Origin	Meaning	Similiar Names
Kasa	Hopi Indian	Fur-robe dress	
Kaya	Hopi Indian	My elder sister-little	
Mansi	Hopi Indian	Plucked flower	

Hungarian Female Baby Names

Name	Origin	Meaning	Similiar Names
Aliz	Hungarian	Kind	
Ildiko	Hungarian	A fierce warrior	
Ilona	Hungarian	Beautiful, sunshine	Ilonka, Ily
Jolan	Hungarian	Violet blossom	Jolanta
Zigana	Hungarian	Gypsy girl	
Zizi	Hungarian	Dedicated to God	
Zsa Zsa	Hungarian	Rose, lilly	Zsusanna, Zsuzsanna, Zuzanny

Indian Female Baby Names

Name	Origin	Meaning	Similiar Names
Ayiana	American Indian	Eternal bloom	
Helki	Miwok Indian	To touch	
Kaliska	Miwok Indian	Coyote chasing deer	
Kasa	Hopi Indian	Fur-robe dress	
Kaya	Hopi Indian	My elder sister-little	
Malila	Miwok Indian	Salmon going fast upstream	
Mansi	Hopi Indian	Plucked flower	
Migina	Omaha Indian	Moon returning	
Natane	Arapaho Indian	Daughter	
Nirvelli	Tudas Indian	Water child	
Orenda	Iroquois Indian	Magic power	
Pakuna	Miwok Indian	Deer jumping down hill	
Poloma	Choctaw Indian	Bow	
Taci	Zuni Indian	Washtub	
Taipa	Miwok Indian	To spread wings	
Talasi	Hopi Indian	Corn-tassel flower	
Tallulah	Choctaw Indian	Leaping water	
Tiponya	Miwok Indian	Owl poking the hatching egg	
Yenene	Miwok Indian	Wizard poisoning a sleeping person	

Irish Female Baby Names

Name	Origin	Meaning	Similiar Names
Akaisha	Irish	The akaisha flower	Casey, Kasey
Ciannait	Irish	Ancient	
Ciar	Irish	Saint's name	Ciara, Cierra
Gale	Irish	Stranger	
Keara	Irish	From a saint's name	
Liadan	Irish	Grey lady	
Moira	Irish, Celtic	Bitter; great	Maura, Moyra
Muriel	Greek, Irish, Latin	Myrrh; sea-bright; angel of June	Murial, Meriel, Muireall
Shanessa	Irish	God is gracious	Nessa
Shannon	Irish	Wise one, river name	Shan, Shanon, Shanen
Sheena	Irish	God's gracious gift	
Sinead	Irish	Gracious	Siobhan

Italian Female Baby Names

Name	Origin	Meaning	Similiar Names
Andria	Italian	Love, joy	Andreea
Bambi	Italian	Child	
Belinda	Spanish, Italian	Beautiful snake	Belynda, Belle, Linda, Blinda
Belladonna	Italian	Beautiful woman	Bella, Bel
Bianca	Italian	White	Biancha, Blanche, Blancha, Blanca
Caprice	Italian	Fanciful, unpredictable	
Carina	Latin, Italian	A keel, beloved, dear	Karina, Caryn, Carynn
Delanna	Italian	Soft as wool	Delana
Donata	Italian	Gift from God	
Donna	Italian	Lady	Dona, Domina, Madonna
Esta	Italian	From the east	
Farfalla	Italian	Butterfly	Farfa, Faffa, Fafylena, Lena, Lina, Faffelina, Lyna, Fafelyna, Fafelina
Fiorenza	Italian	Flower	
Giacinta	Italian	Hyacinth	
Gianina	Italian	God is gracious	
Mariabella	Italian	My beautiful Mary	Mariabelle, Maribel, Maribelle
Mia	Italian	Mine	
Mona	Latin, Greek, Gaelic, Italian	Peaceful; individual; noble one; my lady	
Prima	Italian	First one	
Quorra	Italian	Heart	

Romana	Italian	From Rome	Romy, Roma
Sidonia	Italian	From Sidonia	
Sienna	Italian	Reddish brown	
Tessa	Italian	Countess	
Trilby	Italian	One who sings musical thrills	
Venetia	Italian	From Venice	
Zola	Italian	Ball of earth	

Japanese Female Baby Names

Name	Origin	Meaning	Similiar Names
Ai	Japanese	Love	
Aiko	Japanese	Beloved one, little love	
Akako	Japanese	Red	
Akina	Japanese	Spring flower	
Ami	Japanese	Friend	
Ayame	Japanese	Iris	
Chika	Japanese	Near	
Cho	Japanese	Butterfly	
Dai	Japanese	Great	
Etsu	Japanese	Delight	
Gin	Japanese	Silver	
Gina	Japanese	Silvery	
Hana	Japanese, Hebrew	Flower, blossom; fower, graceful, merciful	
Haya	Japanese	Quick, light	
Hisa	Japanese	Long-lasting	
Iva	Hebrew, Japanese	God's great gift, yew tree	
Jin	Japanese, Korean	Super-excellent; jewel	
Kaede	Japanese	Maple leaf	
Kaiya	Japanese	Forgiveness	
Kameko	Japanese	Tortoise-child, symbol for long-life	
Kaori	Japanese	Fragrant Beautiful Girl	
Kei	Japanese	Rapture, reverence	
Keiko	Japanese	Adored one	
Kichi	Japanese	Fortunate	
Kira	Latin, Persian, Japanese	Light; sun	Keera
Kita	Japanese	North	
Kohana	Japanese	Little flower	
Kyoko	Japanese	Mirror	
Leiko	Japanese	Arrogant	
Machi	Japanese	Ten thousand	
Machiko	Japanese	Child of Machi	
Mai	Japanese, Native American	Brightness; coyote	
Maiko	Japanese	Child of Mai	
Makiko	Japanese	Child of Maki	

Mamiko	Japanese	Child of Mami	
Mariko	Japanese	Child of Mari	
Masako	Japanese	Child of Masa	
Mayako	Japanese	Child of Maya	
Mayoko	Japanese	Child of Mayo	
Mayuko	Japanese	Child of Mayu	
Michi	Japanese	Righteous	
Michiko	Japanese	Child of Michi	
Midori	Japanese	Green	
Mihoko	Japanese	Child of Mihoko	
Mika	Japanese, Finnish	New moon	
Miki	Japanese	Beautiful tree	
Minako	Japanese	Child of Mina	
Mine	Japanese	A resolute protector	
Misako	Japanese	Child of Misa	
Mitsuko	Japanese	Child of Mitsu	
Miyoko	Japanese	Beautiful generations child	
Miyoko	Japanese	Child of Miyo	
Momoko	Japanese	Child of Momo	
Mutsuko	Japanese	Child of Mutsu	
Nahoko	Japanese	Child of Naho	
Nami	Japanese	Wave	
Namiko	Japanese	Child of Nami	
Nanako	Japanese	Child of Nana	
Naoko	Japanese	Child of Nao	
Naomi	Hebrew, Japanese	Pleasent one; above all, beauty	Naoma, Noami, Mimi, Nomi,
Natsuko	Japanese	Child of Natsu	
Nayoko	Japanese	Child of Nayo	
Nori	Japanese	Doctrine	
Noriko	Japanese	Doctrine child	
Noriko	Japanese	Child of Nori	
Nozomi	Japanese	Hope	
Rai	Japanese	Trust	
Rei	Japanese	Gratitude	
Reiko	Japanese	Child of Rei, gratitude	
Ren	Japanese	Water lily	
Rieko	Japanese	Child of Rie	
Rikako	Japanese	Child of Rika	
Rinako	Japanese	Child of Rina	
Rini	Japanese	Little bunny	
Risako	Japanese	Child of Risa	
Ritsuko	Japanese	Child of Ritsu	
Rumiko	Japanese	Child of Rumi	

Ryoko	Japanese	Child of Ryo	
Sachi	Japanese, Hindu	Bliss-child; wife of Indra	
Sachiko	Japanese	Bliss, child of Sachi	
Saeko	Japanese	Child of Sae	
Sakiko	Japanese	Child of Saki	
Sakuko	Japanese	Child of Saku	
Sakura	Japanese	Cherry blossoms	
Sakurako	Japanese	Child of Sakura	
Sanako	Japanese	Child of Sana	
Satoko	Japanese	Child of Sato	
Sayoko	Japanese	Child of Sayo	
Shika	Japanese	Deer	
Shina	Japanese	Virtue, good	
Shoko	Japanese	Child of Sho	
Sorano	Japanese	Of the sky	Sora
Suki	Japanese	Beloved	
Suma	Egyptian, Japanese	To ask	
Sumi	Japanese	Clear, refined	
Tadako	Japanese	Child of Tada	
Taka	Japanese	Tall, honorable	
Takako	Japanese	Child of Taka	
Takara	Japanese	Treasure, precious object	
Tamiko	Japanese	Child of Tami	
Tanaka	Japanese	Dweller	
Tani	Japanese, Melanesian, Tonkinese, Andalusian	Valley; sweetheart; youth; bull that charges randomly	
Tokiko	Japanese	Child of Toki	
Tomiko	Japanese	Child of Tomi	
Tori	Japanese	Bird	
Uma	Hebrew, Hindu, Japanese	Nation, mother, horse	
Usagi	Japanese	Moon	Usa
Yayoi	Japanese	March	
Yoko	Japanese	Positive	
Yoshiko	Japanese	Child of Yoshi	
Yukako	Japanese	Child of Yuka	
Yukiko	Japanese	Child of Yuki	
Yumako	Japanese	Child of Yuma	
Yumi	Japanese	Beauty	
Yumiko	Japanese	Child of Yumi	
Yuri	Japanese	Lily	
Yuriko	Japanese	Child of Yuri	
Yutsuko	Japanese	Child of Yutso	

Korean Female Baby Names

Name	Origin	Meaning	Similiar Names
Bo-Bae	Korean	Treasure, precious	
Dae	Korean	Greatness	
Hea	Korean	Grace	
Hei	Korean	Grace	
Hye	Korean	Graceful	
Hyun	Korean	Wisdom	
Kyung-So	Korean	Honarable, Gentle	
Jin	Japanese, Korean	Super-excellent; jewel	
Joo-Eun	Korean	Silver pearl	
Min	Korean	Cleverness	
Moon	Korean	Letters	
SeaJin	Korean	Jewel of the Universe	
Shin	Korean	Belief	
Sook	Korean	Pure	
Soo	Korean	Excellence, long-life	
Sun	Korean	Goodness	
Sun-Hi	Korean	Goodness,Obedient,Joyful	
Yon	Korean	Lotus Blossom	
Yong	Korean	Courageous, Valiant	
Young	Korean	Eternal Wealth	

Latin Female Baby Names

Name	Origin	Meaning	Similiar Names
Abby	Latin	Head of a monastery	Abbey, Abbe, Abbie
Abigail	Latin, Hebrew	Head of a monastery, a father's joy	Abbey, Abbe, Abbie, Abby, Abagail, Abigayle, Abigale, Gail, Abilio, Abihail
Accalia	Latin	Foster mother of Romulus and Remus	
Adelaide	Hebrew, Latin	Noble, kind, adorned	Adalia, Adeline, Alinc, Adclc, Ellie, Addie, Elle, Adelle, Della, Adailia, Adalee, Adara, Adah, Eda, Etta, Ady, Adela, Adalheld
Adrienne	Greek, Latin	Rich, wealthy, dark one	Adria, Adrea, Adriana, Adrianna, Adrianne, Adreena, Hatria, Adri, Age
Afra	Latin	From Africa	Afraate, Africana
Agnes	Latin, Greek	Lamb, pure, chaste	Agnese, Agnesa, Aggie, Aggy, Agenta, Inez, Ines, Nessa, Neza, Ynes, Ynez, Annice, Annis
Aimee	Latin	Beloved, liked	Amie, Aims, Aimelyn, Aimelin
Akilina	Latin	Eagle	
Albinka	Latin	Blond	

Alida	Greek, Latin	Beautiful dressed, small winged one	Aleda, Aletta, Alette, Allida, Allidia, Alidia, Lida
Allegra	Latin	Brisk and cheerful, full of energy	Allston
Alma	Latin	Soul, nourishing	
Alula	Latin	Winged one	
Alvita	Latin	Anointed, lively	
Amabel	Latin	Lovable	
Amadis	Latin	Love of God	
Amanda	Latin	Love, worthy of love, precious thing	Mandy, Mandie, Mandi
Amandine	Latin	Beloved	
Amdis	Latin	Immortal	
Amelia	Latin	Flatterer, work of the Lord, beloved	Ameilie, Amalia, Amela, Amala, Emelia, Aimee, Amia, Amity, Emele
Ames	Latin	Loves	
Aminta	Latin	Protectress	
Amity	Latin	Friendship	
Amy	Latin	Beloved	
Anabelle	Latin	Lovable	Anabel, Annabel, Ann, Anna, Belle, Bella, Annabelle, Annabella
Ancelin	Latin	Handmaiden	
Andreana	Latin	Womanly	Andrea, Andie, Andy
Annora	Latin	Honor	
Antonia	Latin, Greek	Priceless, flourishing, flower	Antoine, Antoinette, Antoinetta, Antonella, Antonellina, Tonia, Tonya, Toinette, Toni, Tony
April	Latin	Blooming, opening	Avril, Aprille, Ava, Apryl
Araceli	Latin	Alter of heaven	
Ardelia	Latin	Zealous	
Ardere	Latin	Fire	

Ardis	Latin	Fervent	
Aria	Latin	Beautiful melody	Arie, Ariah
Ariadne	Greek, Latin	Melody, very holy one	Ariana, Arianne, Arianna, Ariyaunna, Aria, Ari, Rianna
Arista	Latin	Harvest	
Armina	Latin	Of a high degree	
Aurelia	Latin	Gold	Aurea, Aurelie, Aurilia
Aurora	Latin	Dawn	Aurore
Autumn	Latin	Autumn	
Azadeh	Latin, Persian	Dry earth; detached, free of material things	Ozzie, Oz, Az, Azzie
Balbina	Latin	Strong, stammers	
Barbara	Greek, Latin	Foreign, strange, exotic, mysterious	Barbra, Bararella, Barbie, Barby, Barbs, Barb, Babette, Babs, Bobbie, Bärbel
Beata	Latin, Polish	divinely blessed	Beate
Beatrice	Latin	Happy, bringer of joy	Beatrix, Bea, Beah, Beattie, Beatirsa, Beatriz, Trixie, Trixy
Benita	Latin	Blessed	Bente
Briony	Latin	Plant name	
Brittany	Latin	From England, strong, industrious	Brita, Britta, Brittny, Britannia, Britany, Brit, Britt, Brittyn, Brits, Britney, Britny
Cadence	Latin	Melodious, to fall	
Caledonia	Latin	From Scotland	
Calida	Latin, Spanish	Ardent, warm and loving	
Caltha	Latin	Yellow flower	
Camelai	Latin	Flower name	

Camille	Latin	Attendant at a religious ceremony	Camilla, Camila, Camelia, Cammilla, Cammie, Cammy, Kamilla, Kamille, Mila
Candida	Latin	White, pure	
Candra	Latin	Luminous	
Cara	Latin, Vietnamese	Dear, diamond	Kara, Carra, Karra
Carew	Latin	Run	Carrie, Carry, Cary, Rew
Carha	Latin	A pillar stone	
Carina	Latin, Italian	A keel, beloved, dear	Karina, Caryn, Carynn
Carly	Latin	Little, womanly	Carleen, Karlie, Karly, Karleen, Karlene, Carlene
Carmen	Hebrew, Latin	Garden, field of fruit, song	Carmel, Karmen, Karmel, Carmelita, Karmelita, Carmelle, Karmelle, Carmine, Carmita
Carnelian	Latin	A red gem	
Casilda	Latin	Of the home	
Cassiel	Latin	Angel of saturday, the earthy mother	
Cecilia	Latin	Blind	Cecil, Cecelia, Celia, Cecily, Cicely, Cissy, Sissy, Cicilie, Cece
Celeste	Latin	Heavenly	Celestina, Sally, Chelli, Chelina, Tina
Cerelia	Latin	Of the spring	
Charity	Latin	Affection, charity, brotherly love	
Chastity	Latin	Purity	

Chiara	Latin	Famous, light	Chiarina, Ciaira
Christabel	Latin	Beautiful Christian	
Claire	Latin, Greek	Bright, shining, clear	Clare, Clara, Clarice, Clarissa, Claris, Clarisse, Clarrie, Chiara, Clareta, Clarette, Claretta, Claral, Clairese
Claude	Latin	Lame	Claud, Claudius, Claudell, Claudia, Claudette, Claudio, Klaudia
Clementine	Latin	Merciful	Clementine, Clementyne, Clementina
Constance	Latin	Faithful, firmness	Connie, Constantia, Constanza, Constantine, Constant, Costanza, Konstanzia, Konstanza
Coral	Latin	Rock	
Cordelia	Latin, Celtic	Rope, heart, a sea jewel	Delia, Cordy, Kordelia
Cornelia	Latin	Horn	
Crystal	Latin	Clear, bright, ice	Chrystal, Chrystol, Christal, Krystal, Kristal, Cristal, Cristale, Cristol, Cristel
Cybele	Latin	Prophetess	Cybil, Cybill
Cytheria	Latin	Venus	
Dabria	Latin	Name of an angel	
Dacia	Latin	From Dacia, near Rome	
Daisy	Latin, Old English	Day's eye, flower name	Daisey

Deanna	Latin, Old English	Presiding official, valley	Deane, Deanna, Deana, Deanne, Deena
Delicia	Latin	Delightful one	
Desiree	Latin, French	So long hoped for, crave, desire	Desi, Desideria, Desirae, Desiri
Diana	Latin	Divine	Diane, Dyan, Dyanne, Dionne, Diahann, Di, Diandra, Diantha, Deandra
Diella	Latin	Worships god	
Dillian	Latin	Worshipped one	
Dolores	Latin	Lady of sorrows, from the Virgin Mary	Deloris, Dorrie, Dora, Addolorata, Delores
Elysia	Latin	Sweetly blissful	
Emalia	Latin	Flirt	
Emily	Old German/Latin	Industrious, eager	Emilie, Emelie, Emilia, Emelia, Emiline, Emaline, Emmeline, Emmaline, Emyln, Emelyn, Emmilyne, Em
Esme	Latin	Esteem	Esmee, Esma, Esmie
Estelle	Persian/Latin	Star	Esther, Ester, Estralita, Estel, Estella, Stella, Estie, Estee, Esta, Essie
Eustacia	Latin	Tranquil	Stace, Stacie
Fabiana	Latin	Bean	Fabia, Fabya, Fabienne
Faith	Latin	Trust, faith	Faithful, Faythe, Fayth
Farrah	English, Latin	Beautiful, wild ass	Farah, Farra

Fascienne	Latin	Black	
Fawne	Old French, Latin	Young deer	Fawn, Faun, Fauna, Fawna
Felicia	Latin	Happy	Felice, Felicity, Felisse, Feliciana, Felyce, Phylice, Philicia, Phylicia
Feronia	Latin	Goddess of springs and woods	
Flavia	Latin	Blond, golden hair	Favel
Florence	Latin	Blooming flower, flourishing	Flora, Floria, Florida, Florie, Floris, Florrie, Fleur, Flower, Florenz, Florentia, Flory, Floryn, Flossie, Flo
Florian	Latin	Flowering	
Frances	Latin, Old French	From France, free	Fanchon, Francesca, Fran, Franny, Fanny, Frannie, Francine, Franchesca
Fuscienne	Latin	Black	
Gemma	Latin	Jewel	Jemma
Gillian	Latin	Downy-haired	
Ginger	Latin	Ginger plant	
Gloria	Latin	Glory	
Grace	Latin	Grace, blessing	Grazia, Graziana
Hilary	Latin	Cheerful	Hillary
Honora	Latin	Honor	Honoria
Ilaria	Latin	One who is merry	
Imogene	Latin	Image	
Jinx	Latin	A charm	
Jocelyn	Latin	Happy, joyful	Joceline, Gosceline, Joce
Jocosa	Latin	Gleeful	
Joyce	Latin	Rejoicing	

Julia	Latin	Softhaired, youthful, downy-haired, gentle	Julianne, Julianna, Julie, July, Jules, Juliet
Julinka	Latin	Youthful	Julita
June	Latin	Name of a month	
Justine	Hebrew, Latin	Just, true	Justina, Giustina
Kalare	Latin	Bright, clear	
Kira	Latin, Persian, Japanese	Light; sun	Keera
Kristen	Latin	Follower of Christ	
Lalo	Latin	To sing a lullaby	
Lara	Latin	Well-known, name of a nymph	
Laraine	Latin	Sea bird	
Latonia	Latin	Mother of Apollo and Diana	
Laura	Latin	Laurel leaves, honour, fame, spirit	Laure, Lora, Lori, Lorna, Laurie, Lorry, Laurel, Lauren, Lauryn, Lorin, Laurin, Laurien, Loryn, Laureen, Lauranne, Laurena, Lauretta, Laurette, Lorina, Lorene, Lauriette, Loretta, Lorette, Lorita, Lorenza, Lor
Laurinda	Latin	Crowned with laurel, praise	
Laveda	Latin	Innocent one	Levita
Lavinia	Latin	Purity	Lavine, Lavin
Lena	Latin, Greek	Alluring, temptress; light	Lina, Lenore, Leonore, Leonora, Leonne
Leola	Latin	Lion	Leonarda, Leontine, Leontyne, Leona

Letitia	Latin	Joy	Leticia, Letice, Letizia, Letycia, Leetice, Leta, Letty, Ticia, Tish, Latasha, Laetitia, Laticia
Levana	Latin	Rising sun	
Liana	French, Latin	Vine, to bind; youth	Lianna, Lianne, Liane, Leana
Lily	Latin	A flower	Lilian, Lily Ann, Lilian, Lilianne, Liliana, Lilias, Lilly, Lili, Lilia, Lil, Lis
Lucinda	Latin	Bringer of light	Lucinda, Lucinde, Lukene
Lucretia	Latin	Riches	Lucrezia, Lucrece, Lucy
Lucy	Latin	Light	Lucie, Lucia, Luce, Lou, Lu, Luza, Luz, Luciana, Lucianna, Lucianne, Lucienne, Lucida, Lucile, Lucille, Lucette
Luna	Latin	Moon	Lune, Lunetta
Lupe	Latin	Wolf	
Mabel	French, Latin	My fair maid; lovely	Maybelle, Mabel, Maibelle, Mabella, Maybelline, Mabry, Amabel
Maeve	Greek, Latin	Goddess; a purple flower	
Magna	Latin	Large	Magnilda
Maia	Greek, Latin	Nurse, mother, goddess of spring; great	
Manda	Latin, Hindu	Lovable, harmony; Saturn, God of the occult	

Marcella	Latin, French	God of war; little hammer	Marcy, Marcie, Marcelle, Marceline, Marclyn, Marcelin, Marciana
Marcia	Latin	Martial	Marzia, Marsha, Marshe, Marcille, Marchita, Marchette, Marquita, Martia, Marcelia, Marcy, Marci, Marcie, Marcey, Marsi, Marsy, Marsie
Maren	Latin	Sea	
Margaret	Persian, Latin	Child of light; pearl	Maggie, Maggy, Magee, Mag, Margery, Margareta, Margarita, Margita, Margory, Marjorie, Marjory, Marget, Margret, Margette, Marguerite, Margarida, Margiad, Margherita, Margarethe, Maergrethe, Margaretha, Margalith, Mairghread, Margo, Marjoe, Marga, Margot, Margaux, Marge, Margie, Marta, Madge, Mamie, Maymie, Maisie, Meg, Meggie, Midge, Gretchen, Gretel, Gretle, Greta, Grete, Garet, Peg, Peggy, Rita

Maricel	Latin	Full of grace	Mar, Maricelle
Marissa	Latin	Of the sea	Marisa, Maris, Mari, Marina, Maressa, Maritza, Merisa, Merrisa, Marissah, Rissa
Martina	Latin	Warlike	Marta, Martine, Marty, Tina, Martine
Maura	Latin	Dark	
Maureen	Latin, Gaelic, Old French	Great; little Mary; dark-haired	May, Maura, Mora, Moira, Moreen, Moria, Moriah, Maurin, Maurine, Morena, Maurizia, Mo
Medea	Greek, Latin	Ruling; middle child	Medora, Media, Madora
Mei	Latin	Great one	
Melba	Greek, Latin	Slender, soft; mallow flower	Melva, Malva
Melina	Latin	Canary-yellow	
Mercedes	Latin, Spanish	Ransom; virgin Mary	Mercia, Mercy
Merit	Latin	Deserving	Merritt, Merriwell
Merle	Latin	Blackbird	Merl, Myrle, Meryl, Merlina, Myrlene, Merola, Merrill, Merla
Messina	Latin	Middle child	Messena
Meta	Latin	Ambitious	
Minerva	Greek, Latin	Power; thinker	Minette, Minnie, Minny
Mira	Latin, Spanish; Hebrew	Wonder; aim; light of God	Myra, Mirila, Mirella, Mirelle, Mirielle, Myrilla

Mirabelle	Latin, Spanish	Wonderful; beautiful to look upon	Mirabel, Mrabella, Mirable, Marabel
Miranda	Latin	Extraordinary, to be admired	Myranda, Meranda, Mira, Randy, Mandy
Modestus	Latin	Modest one	
Modesty	Latin	Modest one	Modesta, Modestia, Modestine, Modeste, Desty
Mona	Latin, Greek, Gaelic, Italian	Peaceful; individual; noble one; my lady	
Monica	Latin	Advice	Monca, Mona, Monique
Muriel	Greek, Irish, Latin	Myrrh; sea-bright; Angel of June	Murial, Meriel, Muireall
Myra	Latin, French	Wonderful; quiet song	
Napea	Latin	Of the valley	
Narda	Latin	Fervently anointed	
Natalie	Latin	Birthday, child born at Christmas	Nataly, Natalee, Nataleigh, Natalia, Natalya, Natala, Nataline, Nathalia, Nathalie, Noel, Noelle, Novella, Natasha, Natosha, Natashi, Tosha, Tosh, Natasa, Natashia, Natalja, Natassia, Nastassia, Natividad, Netty, Nettie, Natty, Tally, Tallie, Tasha, Talia
Neci	Latin	Intense, fiery	
Nerissa	Latin	Daughter of the sea	

Nevada	Latin	Snowy	
Nora	Greek, Latin	The bright one; honor, light	Norah, Norine, Noreen, Norina
Norma	Latin	Model	
Nova	Latin	New	Novia
Nydia	Latin	Refuge, nest	
Octavia	Latin	Eighth child	Octavie
Olive	Old Norse, Latin, Old French	Kind one; olive tree, peace	Olivia, Olivya, Olivette, Ollie, Olly, Olva, Livia, Livy, Liv, Livvy, Nollie, Nola
Oona	Gaelic, Latin	Unity	Ona, Oonaugh, Oonagh
Oralia	Latin, Hebrew	Golden; light	Orel, Orelda, Oriole, Orlene, Orlena, Orpah, Oralee, Oralie, Oral, Ora, Orah, Oria, Orlie, Orly, Orabel
Oriana	Latin, Greek	Dawn; east	Oralia, Orelle, Orlanna, Oria
Orianna	Latin	Golden, dawning	Orienne
Oriole	Latin	Fair-haired	
Orla	Latin	Golden woman	
Orlanda	Latin	Bright sun	Orlie
Ortensia	Latin	Gardener, farmer	Hortense
Pantxike	Latin	Free	
Panya	Latin, Swahili	Crowned with laurel; mouse, small child	
Patience	Latin	Suffering	Patty, Patsy, Pat
Patricia	Latin	Noble one	Patrice, Patrizia, Patsy, Patty, Pattie, Patia, Pat, Tricia, Trish, Tish, Rickie, Ricky

Paula	Latin	Petite	Pauline, Paulette, Paulina, Paulita, Paolina, Paola, Pauly, Polly, Pavla, Pavlina, Payne, Pabla
Perdita	Latin	Lost	Perdea, Perda
Peregrine	Latin	Wanderer	
Petra	Latin	Rock, stone	Petronia, Petronella, Petronilla, Pierette, Perrine, Petronille, Petrina, Petrine, Pete, Petie, Pernille
Petula	Latin	Impatient	
Petunia	Latin	A flower	
Placida	Latin	Tranquility	
Portia	Latin	A gift,offering	Porsha, Porsche
Priscilla	Latin	From ancient times	Priss, Prissy, Prisca, Silla, Cilla, Cyla
Prudence	Latin	Foresight	Prudy, Prue, Pru
Prunella	Latin	Little plum	
Quintessa	Latin	Essence	Quintessenz, Quinn, Tess, Tessa
Quintina	Latin	Fifth	Quinta
Quirita	Latin	Citizen	
Rain	Latin	Ruler	Raine, Rein, Reign, Raine, Rayne, Rana, Rane, Raina, Ray, Rain

Regina	Latin	Queenly	Reggie, Gina, Rina, Regan, Reyna, Reine, Rein, Reina, Rain, Rane, Reyna, Rani, Raina, Rexy
Renata	Latin	Reborn	Renate, Renée, Renette
Renita	Latin	To be firm	
Rhea	Greek, Latin	Stream, mother; poppy	Ria, Rea
Risa	Latin	Laughing one	Risë, Risé
Rosanne	Latin	Gracious rose	Rosanna
Rose	Latin, Greek	A flower	Rosa, Rosie, Rosey, Roz, Rozsi, Rosalie, Rosalee, Rosalia, Rosctta, Rosette, Rosina, Rosena, Rasia, Rois, Rosita, Rosebud, Rosabell, Rosly, Roslin, Rosamund, Rosmund, Rosemonde, Rozamund, Roanee, Roanna, Rosaleen, Rosellen, Roselle, Rosella, Rosemary, Rosemarie, Chara, Charo
Rue	Latin, Greek	A herb name; regret	
Sabina	Latin	Sabine woman	Sabine, Savina, Saidhbhin, Sabiny, Biene, Bini, Bienchen, Sabse
Sabrina	Latin	From the border land	Sabrena
Salina	Latin, French	By the salt water; solemn	Saleena

Samara	Hebrew, Latin	Mountain, outlook, ruled by God, guarded by God; seedling	
Sancia	Latin	Holy	
Saxon	Latin, English	Large stone; swordsman	
Scota	Latin	An Irish woman	
Season	Latin	Planting time	
Sebastianne	Latin	Revered one	Sebastiana, Sebastiane, Sebastiona
Semele	Latin	Once	
Septima	Latin	Seventh born	Seven
Serena	Latin	Peaceful one, calm	Serene, Serenity
Sheila	Latin	Blind	Sheilah, Sheela, Sheelah, Selia, Sheilagh
Sidra	Latin	Like a star	
Sileas	Latin	Youth	
Silvia	Latin	Woodland maid	Sylvia, Silva, Silvie, Sylvie, Sylva, Silvana, Sylvana, Sylwia, Zilvia
Solace	Latin	Comfort	
Solita	Latin	Alone	
Spica	Latin	Name of a star	
Stella	Greek, Latin	A star	Stela, Stellar, Star, Starr, Starla, Starling
Tacita	Latin	To be silent	
Tavia	Latin, Old English	Great	Tay, Taves, Tay
Terena	Latin	Earthly	Terrena, Terenna, Terrenna
Terra	Latin	Earth	Terry, Tera
Tertia	Latin	The third	
Tiara	Greek, Latin	Turban, flower name	Teara
Topaz	Latin	Yellow gemstone	
Tosia	Latin	Inestimable	
Trinity	Latin	The holy three	Trin, Triny, Triniti
Trista	Latin	Sorrowful	

Tryphena	Latin	Dainty	
Ultima	Latin	Aloof	
Una	Latin	One, unity, wholeness	Oona
Undine	Latin	Of the wave	Unda, Onde, Ondine
Urbana	Latin	From the citiy	
Ursula	Latin	Little bear	Ursola, Ursule, Orsola, Ursa, Ursie, Orsa, Urzula
Valencia	Latin	Bravery	
Valentine	Latin	Good health	Valentina, Valeda, Valina, Vally, Val, Valtina, Valentiane
Valerie	Old French, Latin	Valor, strong	Valeria, Valery, Valerian, Vally, Vallie, Val, Valarie, Vallerie
Valonia	Latin	Of the vale	
Valora	Latin	The valorous	
Vera	Latin, Slavic	Truth, faith	Verena, Verin, Verina,Verine, Verenia, Vere, Verouska
Veronica	Latin	True image	Veronique, Ronnie, Ron, Nica, Nicky, Ronica
Vesper	Latin	Evening	Vespera
Vesta	Latin	Guardian of the sacred fire	
Vevina	Latin	Sweet lady	
Victoria	Latin	Victory	Vicki, Vicky, Viktoria, Vitoria, Victoire, Victory, Vickie, Vic, Toria, Torey, Torri, Tori, Victorienne
Vidonia	Latin	Vine branch	
Vienna	Latin	From wine country	
Violet	Latin	Violet	Viola

Virginia	Latin	Chaste, maiden	Virginie, Virgie, Virgy, Gina, Ginia, Ginny, Ginni, Ginger, Jinny
Viridis	Latin	Youthful and blooming	
Vita	Latin	Life	Vitas, Verta, Vitia
Vivian	Latin	Living, lively	Vivien, Vivianne, Viviana, Vivienne, Vyvyan, Vivyen, Vivyan, Viviana, Vivie, Viv, Vibiana, Viveca
Zama	Latin	Came from Zama	
Zia	Hebrew, Latin	To tremble, a kind of grain	
Zona	Latin	Prostitute	

Native American Female Baby Names

Name	Origin	Meaning	Similiar Names
Abey	Native American	Leaf	
Aiyana	Native American	Eternal bloom	Ajana
Alaqua	Native American	Sweet-gum tree	
Aleshanee	Native American	She plays all the time	
Alona	Native American	Oak tree	
Amitola	Native American	Rainbow	
Angeni	Native American	Spirit angel	
Aponi	Native American	Butterfly	
Aquene	Native American	Peace	
Ayita	Native American	Worker	
Benquasha	Native American	Daughter of Ben	Quasha, Quay
Bly	Native American	High, tall	
Chenoa	Native American	White dove	
Chilali	Native American	Snowbird	
Chimalis	Native American	Bluebird	
Dena	Hebrew, Native American	Vindicated, valley	Denna
Dyani	Native American	Deer	
Enola	Native American	Magnolia	
Etania	Native American	Wealthy	
Eyota	Native american	Greatest one	
Fala	Native American	Crow	
Halona	Native American	Fortunate	
Huyana	Native American	Rain falling	
Istas	Native American	Snow	
Kachine	Native American	Sacred dancer	Kachina
Kiona	Native American	Brown hills	
Koko	Native American	Night	
Magena	Native American, Hebrew	The coming moon; a covering, protection	
Mahala	Native American, Hebrew, Arabic	Woman; tenderness; marrow	Mahalah, Mahalar, Mahela, Mahalia, Mahelia, Mehala
Mai	Japanese, Native American	Brightness; coyote	

Meda	Native American	Priestess	
Miakoda	Native American	Power of the moon	
Minda	Native American	Knowledge	
Mitena	Native American	Coming moon, new moon	
Mitexi	Native American	Sacred moon	
Nara	Old English, Gaelic, Native A	Near one; joyous; place name	
Nita	Native American	Bear	
Nitika	Native American	Angel of precious stone	
Olathe	Native American	Beautiful	
Onida	Native American	The expected one	
Sakari	Native American	Sweet	
Satinka	Native American	Magic dancer	
Shako	Native American	Mint	
Shysie	Native American	Silent little one	
Taborri	Native American	Voices that carry	Taborah, Tabby
Tacincala	Native American	Deer	Tawi
Taima	Native American	Crash of thunder	
Tainn	Native American	New moon	
Takoda	Native American	Friend to all	
Tala	Native American	Stalking wolf	
Tama	Native American	Thunderbolt	Tamah
Tareva-Chine(shanay)	Native American	Beautiful eyes	Tu-Sha
Tayen	Native American	New moon	
Tehya	Native American	Precious	
Waneta	Native American	Charger	
Wapeka	Native American	Skillful	
Winema	Native American	Female chief	
Zaltana	Native American	High mountain	

Nigerian Female Baby Names

Name	Origin	Meaning	Similiar Names
Akanke	Nigerian	To know her is to love her	
Alike	Nigerian	Girl who drives out beautiful women	
Bayo	Nigerian	To find joy	
Sade	Nigerian	Honor confers a crown	

Norse Female Baby Names

Name	Origin	Meaning	Similiar Names
Astrid	Greek, Old Norse	Star, super strength, divine strength	Astera, Astred, Asta, Astyr
Erika	Old Norse, Old English, Old German	Ever-powerful	Erica, Eryka, Ericka, Enrica
Flos	Norse	Chieftain	
Haldis	Teutonic, Norse	Stone spirit; reliable, assistant	
Nessa	Old Norse	Headland	Nesa, Nissa, Nessie
Oda	Norse	Small pointed spear	
Olive	Old Norse, Latin, Old French	Kind one; olive tree, peace	Olivia, Olivya, Olivette, Ollie, Olly, Olva, Livia, Livy, Liv, Livvy, Nollie, Nola
Ragnhild	Norse	One who is wise in battle	
Ronalda	Old Norse	Mighty	
Sigrid	Old Norse	Winning adviser	Sigrath, Sigwald, Sigurd
Thora	Old Norse	Thunder	Thordia, Tora
Valda	Old Norse	Spirited warrior	

Norwegian Female Baby Names

Name	Origin	Meaning	Similiar Names
Andras	Norwegian	Breath	
Aundy	Norwegian	New prosperity	
Birget	Norwegian	Protecting	
Borgny	Norwegian	Help, new	
Bryn	Welsh, Norwegian	Hill, coat	Brynn
Dagny	Norwegian	Day, brightness, new day, Dane's joy	
Disa	Norwegian	Active spirit	
Freya	Norwegian	Noble woman, Godess of love and Seduction	Freia
Lene	Norwegian	Illustrious	
Linnea	Norwegian	Lime tree, national flower of Sweden	
Liv	Norwegian	Life	
Rane	Norwegian	Queen, pure	
Reidun	Norwegian	Nest-lovely	
Siv	Norwegian	Kinship, wife of Thor	Seev

Persian Female Baby Names

Name	Origin	Meaning	Similiar Names
Azadeh	Latin, Persian	Dry earth; detached, free of material things	Ozzie, Oz, Az, Azzie
Azura	Persian	Sky-blue	Azure
Dara	Hebrew, Persian	Compassion, wisdom, angel of rains and rivers	
Daria	Persian	Queen	Darine
Estelle	Persian/Latin	Star	Esther, Ester, Estralita, Estel, Estella, Stella, Estie, Estee, Esta, Essie
Gelsey	Persian	A flower	Gelsi, Gelsy
Jasmine	Persian	Jasmine flower, gift from God	Jasmin, Yasmin, Yasmine, Jessamine, Jessamy, Jess, Yazmina, Mine, Mina
Kira	Latin, Persian, Japanese	Light; sun	Keera

Margaret	Persian, Latin	Child of light; pearl	Maggie, Maggy, Magee, Mag, Margery, Margareta, Margarita, Margita, Margory, Marjorie, Marjory, Marget, Margette, Marguerite, Margarida, Margherita, Margarethe, Margaretha, Margo, Margot, Marge, Margie, Marta, Madge, Mamie, Maisie, Meg, Meggie, Gretchen, Gretel, Gretle
Parisa	Persian	Angelic face	
Roxanne	Persian	Brilliant one	Roxane, Roxann, Roxanna, Roxie, Roxy, Rox, Roxana
Vashti	Persian	Beautiful	
Yasmine	Persian	Flowering olive	
Zita	Hebrew, Persian	The seeker; virgin	

Polish Female Baby Names

Name	Origin	Meaning	Similiar Names
Alina	Polish	Bright, beautiful	
Basha	Hebrew, Greek, Polish	Daughter of God, stranger	
Beata	Latin, Polish	Divinely blessed	Beate
Felcia	Polish	Lucky	
Olesia	Polish	Helper and defender of mankind	
Rasine	Polish	A rose	Roisine
Tesia	Polish	Loved by God	
Tola	Polish	Priceless	
Valeska	Polish	Glorious ruler	
Zotia	Polish	One with Wisdom	Zosia

Polynesian Female Baby Names

Name	Origin	Meaning	Similiar Names
Ema	Polynesian	Beloved	
Kaimi	Polynesian	The seeker	
Kaula	Polynesian	Prophet	
Lana	Polynesian	To float	

Russian Female Baby Names

Name	Origin	Meaning	Similiar Names
Bohdana	Russian	From God	Bogdana
Cyzarine	Russian	Royalty	Cyzars
Fayina	Russian	Free one	
Galina	Russian	Light	
Jelena	Russian	Shining light	Yelena, Ielena, Elena, Laney, Lena
Kisa	Russian	Kitty	
Kiska	Russian	Pure	
Larissa	Greek, Russian	Name of a city, mythical woman; cheerful one	
Marina	Russian	Sea maiden	
Nika	Russian	Born on Sunday	
Oksana	Russian	Glory be to God	Oksanochka
Olga	Russian	Holy	
Sashenka	Russian	Defender and helper of mankind	
Sonia	Russian	Wisdom	Sonja, Sonya
Svetlana	Russian	Star	
Tanya	Russian	Fairy princess	Tania, Tan, Tani, Tatiana, Tatjana
Vania	Russian	God's gift	
Vanya	Russian	Gracious gift of God	Wanja, Vanja, Vania, Wania, Wanya
Yeva	Russian	Live-giving	

Sanskrit Female Baby Names

Name	Origin	Meaning	Similiar Names
Chandani	Sanskrit	Name of the goddess Devi	Chandan, Chanda
Chandi	Sanskrit	Angry name of goddess Sakti	
Chandra	Sanskrit	Eminent, illustrious, moon	
Deva	Sanskrit	Divine	
India	Sanskrit, English	River; from India	
Kali	Sanskrit	Energy, dark goddess	
Kalinda	Sanskrit	Sun, name of mountains	Kalin
Kama	Sanskrit	Love	
Manjusha	Sanskrit	A box of jewels	
Nalini	Sanskrit	Lovely	
Opal	Sanskrit	Jewel	
Sitara	Sanskrit	Morning star	
Tamara	Hebrew, Sanskrit	Palm tree, spice	Tamarah, Tamar, Tamarind, Tamika, Tamary

Saxon Female Baby Names

Name	Origin	Meaning	Similiar Names
Alodie	Anglo-Saxon	Wealthy	
Bliss	Anglo-Saxon	Joy	
Capri	Anglo-Saxon	The goat	
Darlene	Anglo-Saxon	Tenderly beloved, little darling	Darlin, Darlen, Darleen, Darlynn, Dare, Darla
Ebba	Germanic/Anglo-Saxon	Strength, return of the tide	
Faina	Anglo-Saxon	Joyful	
Githa	Anglo-Saxon	Gift	
Kendra	Anglo-Saxon	Understaning, knowledge	
Kirby	Anglo-Saxon	From the church town	
Lynn	Anglo-Saxon	A cascade	
Mildred	Anglo-Saxon	Mild, power	Mildrid, Mildraed, Mildryd, Milly, Milli, Milley, Millie, Hildred, Hil, Mil
Walburga	Anglo-Saxon	A mighty defender, a fortress	Walburg

Scandinavian Female Baby Names

Name	Origin	Meaning	Similiar Names
Kelda	Scandinavian	Clear mountain spring	Kelley, Kelly, Kel, Kell
Selma	Scandinavian	Divinely protected	
Nissa	Scandinavian	Elf, fairy	Nisse, Nissi, Nissan, Nissim
Marny	Scandinavian	From the sea	
Haley	Scandinavian	Hero	Hailey
Helga	Scandinavian	Holy, faithful	
Hilda	Scandinavian	Protector	Hilde
Runa	Scandinavian	Secret lore	
Ylwa	Scandinavian	She-wolf	Ylva
Quenby	Scandinavian	Womanly	

Scottish Female Baby Names

Name	Origin	Meaning	Similiar Names
Ainsley	Scottish	My meadow	Aynsley, Ainsly, Ainslee, Ainsworth
Bonnie	Scottish	Sweet and good	Bonny, Boni, Boniface, Bonita
Grear	Scottish	Watchful	
Leslie	Scottish, Old English	Dweller in the gray castle	Lesley, Lesly, Les, Lee
Maisie	Scottish	Child of light	Maisy, Maysie, Mysie, Mazey, Maizie
Manhattan	Old English, Scottish	Whiskey	Manny, Manda, Maisie
Minna	Old German, Scottish, Hebrew	Love; mother; bitterness	Mina, Minette, Minetta, Minda, Myna, Mindy
Vanora	Scottish	White wave	

Slavic Female Baby Names

Name	Origin	Meaning	Similiar Names
Alena	Greek, Slavic	Pretty, light	Olena
Berta	Germanic, Slavic	Glorious, learning	
Chesna	Slavic	Peaceful	
Danica	Slavic	The morning star	
Kamilia	Slavic	Sweet flower	
Kasmira	Old Slavic	Demands peace	Kasamira, Kazamira
Klavdia	Slavic	A lame one	
Lala	Slavic	Tulip	
Nadine	Slavic	Hope	Nada, Nadina, Nadeen, Nadia, Nata, Nadya, Nadie, Nadezhda
Neda	Slavic, English	Born on Sunday; sanctuary	Nedda, Neddy, Ned, Nerida, Nedjelko, Nedo
Radinka	Slavic	Active	
Velika	Slavic	Great	
Vera	Latin, Slavic	Truth, faith	Verena, Verin, Verina,Verine, Verenia, Vere, Verouska
Yarmilla	Slavic	Merchant	
Zora	Slavic, Greek	Golden dawn	Zorah, Zoradah, Zohra, Zarya, Zoranna, Zorina, Zoriana, Zori, Zorie, Zorry

Spanish Female Baby Names

Name	Origin	Meaning	Similiar Names
Adoncia	Spanish	Sweet	
Alita	Spanish	Noble	
Amata	Spanish	Beloved	
Anika	Hindu, Spanish	Very beautiful, graceful	Anica
Arcadia	Spanish	Adventurous	
Belicia	Spanish	Dedicated to God	Isabel, Isabelle
Belinda	Spanish, Italian	Beautiful snake	Belynda, Belle, Linda, Blinda
Calida	Latin, Spanish	Ardent, warm and loving	
Cochiti	Spanish	Forgotten	
Dominga	Spanish	Sunday	Inga
Dorota	Greek, Spanish	God's gift	
Drina	Spanish	Helper and defender of mankind	
Dulcinea	Spanish	Sweet	Dulcie, Dulce, Dulsie, Dolce, Dulcea
Elena	Spanish	The bright one	
Elisa	Spanish	Dedicated to God	Elyse, Lyse, Lysa, Elysa, Elise, Lise, Lisa, Lisie
Elvira	Spanish	Impartial judgement, close	Eli, Elvyra, Elvera, Elvie, Elva
Emerald	Spanish	A bright green gem	Esmeralda, Esmarelda, Esmaralda, Esmiralda, Esmirelda, Esmerelda
Eskarne	Spanish	Merciful	
Esperanza	Spanish	Hope	

Fuensanta	Spanish	A holy fountain	
Gitana	Spanish	Gypsy	
Hermelinda	Spanish	Shield of power	
Herminia	Spanish	Lady of the earth	Minney, Mini
Ines	Spanish	Gentle	
Isabel	Spanish	Concecrated to God	Isabella, Isabelle, Izzy, Sabel
Isleta	Spanish	Little Island	
Jaimica	Spanish	Supplanter	
Kesare	Spanish	Long-haired	
Linda	Spanish	Pretty	Lynda, Lindy, Lindi, Lin, Linden, Belinda
Lola	Spanish	Strong woman	Lolita
Madeira	Spanish	Sweet wine	
Madra	Spanish	Mother	Madre, Madrona
Manuela	Spanish	God is with us	
Mariposa	Spanish	Butterfly	
Melisenda	Spanish	Honest, diligent	
Melosa	Spanish	Gentle, sweet	
Mercedes	Latin, Spanish	Ransom; virgin Mary	Mercia, Mercy
Mira	Latin, Spanish; Hebrew	Wonder; aim; light of God	Myra, Mirila, Mirella, Mirelle, Mirielle, Myrilla
Mirabelle	Latin, Spanish	Wonderful; beautiful to look upon	Mirabel, Mrabella, Mirable, Marabel
Mireya	Spanish	Mircaulous	Mirielle, Mireille
Mora	Spanish	Blueberry	Morella, Morina
Neva	Spanish	Covered with snow	Nevia, Nevea, Nevita
Nina	Spanish, Hebrew	Girl; grace	Ninya, Ninette, Ninon

Paloma	Spanish	Dove	Palometa, Palomita, Palita, Palomita, Palomina
Patia	Spanish	Leaf	
Pilar	Spanish	Pillar	
Raeka	Spanish	Beautiful, unique	Rae
Ramona	Spanish	Wise protector	Ramonda, Mona
Ria	Spanish	Mouth of a river	
Rosalind	Spanish, Teutonic	Pretty rose; horse serpent	Rosalinda, Rosaline, Roseline, Rosalyn, Roselyn, Rosey, Rosilind, Rose-Lyn, Roslin
Sally	Spanish	Saviour	Salaidh, Sallye, Salli, Sallie, Sal
Sandia	Spanish	Watermelon	
Savanna	Old Spanish	From the open plain	Savannah
Sierra	Spanish	Saw-tooth mountain range	
Solana	Spanish	Sunshine	
Soledad	Spanish	Solitary, health	
Tia	Spanish, Greek	Aunt, princess	Tianna, Tiana
Tierra	Spanish	Earth, land	
Xiomara	Spanish	Xiomy	
Yomaris	Spanish	I am the sun	Maris, Marisol

Swahili Female Baby Names

Name	Origin	Meaning	Similiar Names
Aziza	Swahili, Turkish	Precious	Azize, Azy
Barika	Swahili	Bloom	
Binty	Swahili	Daughter	
Jina	Swahili	Name	Gina
Kamaria	Swahili	Like the moon	
Kesi	Swahili	Born when father was in trouble	
Lakeisha	Swahili	Favourite one	Lawanna, Latasha, Latoya, Latonya
Nia	Swahili	Purpose	
Panya	Latin, Swahili	Crowned with laurel; mouse, small child	
Penda	Swahili	Love	
Shani	Swahili	Marvellous	
Simba	Swahili	Lion	
Winda	Swahili	Hunt	
Zahra	Arabic, Swahili	White, flowers	

Swedish Female Baby Names

Name	Origin	Meaning	Similiar Names
Dana	Swedish, Celtic	From Denmark, mother of the Gods in myths	
Gala	Swedish	Singer	
Inga	Swedish	Hero's daughter	Inge
Maj	Swedish	Pearl	
Signe	Swedish	A sign, victorious	
Trind	Swedish	Pure	
Valborg	Swedish	A powerful mountain	

Teutonic Female Baby Names

Name	Origin	Meaning	Similiar Names
Acelin	Teutonic	Noble	
Ada	Teutonic, Hebrew	Happy, ornament	Adah
Aldea	Teutonic	Rich	
Aloysia	Teutonic	Famous in war	
Blanda	Teutonic	Dazzling	Blenda
Carla	Teutonic	One who is strong, woman	Carol, Caroll, Carlotta, Carlota, Karla, Karol, Karola, Carola
Carlen	Teutonic	Woman	
Della	Teutonic	Of nobility	Dell, Adella, Adela
Edith	Teutonic	Rich gift, happy	Edie, Edita, Edythe, Edyth, Edithe, Edda, Editha
Geraldine	Teutonic	Ruler with the spear	Jeri, Gerry, Gery, Geraldina, Geraldene, Gereldine, Geraldyne, Geri, Gerrie

Gertrude	Teutonic	Spear maiden	Gertrud, Gerta, Gerda, Gerte, Gertie, Gerty, Gert, Jera, Jerica, Trude, Truta, Trudy, Trudie, Trudi, True
Gilen	Teutonic	Industrious pledge	
Haldis	Teutonic, Norse	Stone spirit; reliable, assistant	
Henka	Teutonic	Ruler of an estate	
Ingrid	Teutonic	Hero's daughter, a meadow	
Kelly	Gaelic, Teutonic	Church, warrior, wood, holly; farm by the spring	Kel
Magan	Teutonic	Power	
Minka	Teutonic	Strong, resolute	
Orinda	Teutonic	Fire serpent	
Rosalind	Spanish, Teutonic	Pretty rose; horse serpent	Rosalinda, Rosaline, Roseline, Rosalyn, Roselyn, Rosey, Rosilind, Rose-Lyn, Roslin
Verena	Teutonic	Defender	
Waltraud	Teutonic	Rule strength	

Turkish Female Baby Names

Name	Origin	Meaning	Similiar Names
Akasma	Turkish	White climbing-rose	
Aziza	Swahili, Turkish	Precious	Azize, Azy
Cari	Turkish	Flows like water	Kari
Culay	Turkish	Rosemoon	
Fairuza	Turkish	Turquoise	
Gizem	Turkish	Mysterious	
Harika	Turkish	Wonderful	
Irem	Turkish	Gardens in heaven	
Jihan	Turkish	Universe	
Kari	Turkish	Flows like water	Cari, Carrie, Keri, Kery, Kary
Karli	Turkish	Covered with snow	Karlie
Nuray	Turkish	White moon	
Sevilin	Turkish	Beloved	
Sila	Turkish	Homesick	
Zeynep	Turkish	Daughter of the prophet Muhammed	

Ugadan Female Baby Names

Name	Origin	Meaning	Similiar Names
Acanit	Ugandan	Hard times	
Achen	Ugandan	A twin	
Bacia	Ugandan	Family deaths ruined the home	
Dembe	Ugandan	Peace	
Jendyose	Ugandan	Have done good to produce a child	
Kenyangi	Ugandan	White egret	
Kissa	Ugandan	Born after twins	
Miremba	Ugandan	Peace	
Namazzi	Ugandan	Water	
Nantale	Ugandan	Clan totem is a lion	
Nasiche	Ugandan	Born during locust season	

Vietnamese Female Baby Names

Name	Origin	Meaning	Similiar Names
Bian	Vietnamese	Secretive, hidden	
Cara	Latin, Vietnamese	Dear, diamond	Kara, Carra, Karra
Dep	Vietnamese	Beautiful	
Hue	Vietnamese	Lily	
Lan	Vietnamese	Flower name	
My-Duyen	Vietnamese	Beautiful, pretty	
Mychau	Vietnamese	Great	Mah Chow
Nhu	Vietnamese	Everything according to one's wishes	
Tam	Vietnamese	Heart	

Welsh Female Baby Names

Name	Origin	Meaning	Similiar Names
Ariene	Welsh	Silvery	
Bronwyn	Welsh	Fair breast	
Bryn	Welsh, Norwegian	Hill, coat	Brynn
Caitlin	Celtic, Welsh	Pure	Caitlyn, Kaitlin, Kaitlyn, Katelyn, Catelyn, Caitrin
Caradoc	Welsh	Amiable	
Dilys	Welsh	Genuine	
Emlyn	Welsh	Place name	Emlin
Enid	Welsh	Quiet woman, soul	
Glynis	Welsh	Little valley	Glynn, Gwen, Gwyndolyn
Guinevere	Welsh	White, fair; white wave	Gwen
Gwyneth	Welsh	White; blessed, fortunate	Gwynne, Wynny
Jennifer	Welsh	White wave, white spirit, white cheeked	Jenna, Jenny, Jenni, Jennie, Jennylynn, Jenavieva, Vieva, Genavieve
Megan	Greek, Gaelic, Welsh	Mighty, strong able, pearl	Meggy, Meghan, Meagan, Megann, Meggy, Meggie, Meg, Megs, Megless

Morgan	Gaelic, Welsh	White sea; bright, dweller by the sea	Morgana, Morganne, Morganica
Myfanwy	welsh	Sweet woman	
Rhiamon	Welsh	Witch	Rhianon
Rhiannon	Welsh	A mythological nymph	
Riannon	Welsh	Great queen, witch, or goddess	Rianne, Riana
Taffy	Welsh	Beloved	
Vevay	Welsh	White wave	
Wynn	Welsh	Fair	Wynne, Wyn, Wynnie, Winnie, Winny, Win, Winn, Weeny

Yiddish Female Baby Names

Name	Origin	Meaning	Similiar Names
Enye	Yiddish	Grace	
Fruma	Yiddish	One who is religious	
Leba	Yiddish	Beloved	
Mindel	Yiddish	Sea of bitterness	
Shayndel	Yiddish	Beautiful	
Syshe	Yiddish	Street	

Yoruban Female Baby Names

Name	Origin	Meaning	Similiar Names
Abiona	Yoruban	Born on a journey	
Adesina	Yoruban	The way is opened for more	
Aina	Yoruban	Complicated delivery	
Alake	Yoruban	One petted	
Amoke	Yoruban	To pet her	
Apara	Yoruban	One who comes and goes	
Jumoke	Yoruban	Everyone loves the baby	Yumoke
Kehinde	Yoruban	Second of tiwns	
Olayinka	Yoruban	Honors surround me	

Male Baby Names with Meanings and Origins

African Male Baby Names

Name	Origin	Meaning	Similiar Names
Jelani	African	Mighty	
Juma	African	Born on a Friday	
Mablevi	African	Do not deceive	
Nabulung	African	Do not receive	
Naeem	North African	Benevolent	
Obiajulu	African	The heart is consoled	
Razi	African	Secret	
Runako	African	Handsome	
Salim	African	Peace	
Sulaiman	North African	Peaceful	
Tabansi	African	One who endures	
Tabari	North African	After a famous Muslim historian	
Uba	African	Wealthy	
Yobachi	African	Pray to God	
Zaid	African	Increase, growth	
Zabia	African	Unknown	

Anglo-Saxon Male Baby Names

Name	Origin	Meaning	Similiar Names
Aiken	Anglo-Saxon	Sturdy, oaken	
Alston	Anglo-Saxon	From the old manor	Alton
Anson	Anglo-Saxon	Son of a nobleman, son of Ann or Hans	Ansen, Ansonia, Hansen, Hanson
Archibald	Anglo-Saxon	Bold prince	Arch, Archie, Archy, Arkady, Arky
Bardon	Anglo-Saxon	Barley valley	
Berkeley	Anglo-Saxon	From the birch meadow	Berkley
Boyden	Anglo-Saxon	A herald	
Braxton	Anglo-Saxon	Brock's town	
Byron	French, Anglo-Saxon	From the cottage, bear	Byram, Byran
Daley	Gaelic, Anglo-Saxon	Assembly, from the valley	Dailey, Daily
Eamon	Anglo-saxon	Wealthy guardian	Amon
Elvis	Anglo-Saxon	All wise, noble friend	
Garett	Anglo-Saxon	Powerful with the spear	
Graham	Anglo-Saxon	warlike	
Irvin	Anglo-Saxon	Lover of the sea	Irv, Irvine
Marvin	Celtic, Anglo-Saxon	Beautiful sea; good friend	Mervin, Mervyn, Merwin, Merwyn, Myrwyn, Murvyn, Myrvyn, Marv
Maynard	Anglo-Saxon	Remarkable strength	
Melville	Anglo-Saxon, Old English	Hillside; town by the mill	Mel

Merlin	Celtic, Anglo-Saxon, Welsh	Sea; falcon; sea hill	Merlyn, Marlin, Marlen, Marwin, Mervin, Merv, Merle
Morton	Anglo-Saxon	City on the moor	Morten, Mortyn, Morty, Mort
Randolph	Anglo-Saxon	Shield, wolf	Randolf, Randall, Randal, Randell, Randl, Randle, Randy, Rankin, Rand, Ran, Randie, Ranulf, Dolf, Dolph
Ross	Scottish, Anglo-Saxon	From the peninsula; horse	Rossano, Roswald

Arabic Male Baby Names

Name	Origin	Meaning	Similiar Names
Aaron	Hebrew, Arabic	Shining light, high mountain, messenger	Aron, Ahron, Arron
Abbott	Arabic, Aramaic, Hebrew	Father	Abbot, Abba, Abbe, Absa
Abdel	Arabic	Servent	Abdon, Abdone
Akil	Arabic	Intelligent, logical	
Aleser	Arabic	Lion	
Ali	Arabic, Native American	God, little, the highest	Allah
Alim	Arabic	Wise, learned	
Amir	Arabic	Prince	Ameer
Basil	Greek, Arabic	Royal, brave	Basile, Basilo, Basilia, Basia, Vasilis, Vasily
Bilal	Arabic	First convert of Muhammad	
Burhan	Arabic	Proof	
Cemal	Arabic	Beauty	Kemal, Cem
Coman	Arabic	Noble	
Emir	Arabic	Charming prince	
Ferran	Arabic	Baker	
Gadil	Arabic	God is my wealth	
Gamal	Arabic	Camel	Jamal, Jammal, Gamali
Ginton	Arabic	A garden	
Givon	Arabic	Hill, heights	
Habib	Arabic	Beloved one	
Hadi	Arabic	Guiding to the light	
Hamal	Arabic	Lamb	
Hassan	Arabic	Handsome	
Hussein	Arabic	Handsome one	
Jabir	Arabic	Comforter	

Jaleel	Arabic	Great, fine	
Jamal	Arabic	Beauty	
Jed	Arabic	The hand	
Jibril	Arabic	Archangel Gabriel	
Kadin	Arabic	Friend, companion	Kadeen, Kaden
Kalb	Arabic	Dog	
Kalil	Arabic	Good/best friend	Kahill, Kailil, Khalil
Kamil	Arabic	Perfection	Camillo, Kamillo
Kardal	Arabic	Mustard seed	
Kateb	Arabic	Writer	
Khalid	Arabic	Immortal	Khaled
Khoury	Arabic	Priest	
Laith	Arabic	Lion	
Leron	Arabic	The song is mine	
Malik	Arabic	Master	
Mansur	Arabic	Divinely aided	
Muhammad	Arabic	Praised one	Muhammed, Mohamad, Mohammed, Mohamed, Mohammad
Nassir	Arabic	Protector	Nas, Nasir
Nuri	Arabic	Fire	
Omar	Arabic, Hebrew, German	First son, disciple; gifted speaker; famous	Omer
Quasim	Arabic	One who divides goods among his people	
Rimon	Arabic	Pomegranite	
Salman	Arabic	Protector, conqueror	
Samien	Arabic	To be heard	
Sammon	Arabic	Grocer	
Seif	Arabic	Sword of religion	
Shakar	Arabic	Grateful	
Shunnar	Arabic	Pleasant	
Tahir	Arabic	Chaste, pure	
Tamir	Arabic	Pure, tall stately	
Tariq	Arabic	Star, path	Tarik, Taric, Tareeq, Tareek, Tareec
Utt	Arabic	Wise and kind	

Xavier	Arabic, Basque	Bright, new house	Xaver, Xever, Javier
Yasir	Arabic	To be rich, to be easy	
Zeke	Arabic	The memory of the Lord	

Armenian Male Baby Names

Name	Origin	Meaning	Similiar Names
Aram	Armenian	High, Exalted	
Armen	Armenian	Armenian	
Arpiar	Armenian	Sunny	
Arsen	Armenian	Strong, Potent	
Artaxiad	Armenian	King's Name	
Avedis	Armenian	Good News	
Bedros	Armenian	Rock	
Boghos	Armenian	Small, Humble	
Brosh	Armenian	Lips	
Carnig	Armenian	Small Lamb	
Dareh	Armenian	Wealthy One	
Hagop	Armenian	Supplanter, Representative	
Haig	Armenian	Legend, From the field	
Hovan	Armenian	God's Gift	
Hovhannes	Armenian	God is Gracious	
Hovsep	Armenian	God will increase	
Jirair	Armenian	Strong, Hardworking	
Kaloosh	Armenian	Blessed Event	
Keran	Armenian	Wooden Post	
Kevork	Armenian	Farmer	
Khajag	Armenian	Blue eyes	
Kirkan	Armenian	Vigilant, Watchful	
Krikor	Armenian	Vigilant, Watchful	
Levon	Armenian	Lion	
Nishan	Armenian	Sign, Mark	
Phyre	Armenian	Burning Bright	
Sevan	Armenian	Armenian Lake	
Vahan	Armenian	Shield	
Vanig	Armenian	Small Town	
Vartan	Armenian	Giver of Roses	
Yervant	Armenian	Armenian King	

Basque Male Baby Names

Name	Origin	Meaning	Similiar Names
Aita	Basque	Father	
Aitor	Basque	Good Father	
Ander	Basque	Courageous, Valiant Man	
Basajaun	Basque	Forest Lord	
Baso	Basque	Woods	
Enrique	Basque	Ruler of estate	
Etxabier	Basque	Bright, New House	
Eztebe	Basque	Crowned	
Gorka	Basque	Farmer	
Gutxi	Basque	Small	
Ramiro	Basque	Great judge	
Inaki	Basque	Fiery	
Jaun	Basque	Lord	
Jon	Basque	God is Gracious	
Mikel	Basque	Reference to Virgin Mary	
Txomin	Basque	Belonging to God	
Xabier	Basque	Bright New House	
Ximun	Basque	Listener	

Breton Male Baby Names

Name	Origin	Meaning	Similiar Names
Corentin	Breton	Hurricane	
Erwan	Breton	Yew	
Gwilherm	Breton	Desiring Protector	
Haerviu	Breton	Ready for battle	
Jodoc	Breton	Lord	
Loic	Breton	Famous Warrior	
Padrig	Breton	Noble	
Pierreck	Breton	Rock,Powerful ruler	
Viu	Breton	Worthy	
Yanick	Breton	God Is Gracious	Yann, Yannic, Yannick

Celtic Male Baby Names

Name	Origin	Meaning	Similiar Names
Adalardo	Celtic	Noble	Alart, Adelardo
Ahearn	Celtic	Lord of the horses	
Alan	Gaelic, Celtic	Handsome, cheerful, noble	Allen, Allan, Alain, Alano
Amon	Celtic, Egyptian	The hidden	Ammon, Eamon, Eammon, Edmund
Angus	Gaelic, Celtic	Superb, unique	
Arland	Celtic	Pledge	Arles, Arleigh, Arlo, Arly, Arlie, Arlen, Arliss, Arlyss
Arthur	Celtic	Noble, follower of Thor	Arthie, Arty, Arturo, Artu
Barry	French, Celtic, Welsh	Spear thrower, son of Harry, Marksman	Barrie, Barris, Barie, Barrymore
Beacan	Celtic, Gaelic	Small, little one	Beagan
Boyd	Celtic	Blond, yellow	
Bram	Gaelic, Celtic	Raven	
Brazil	Celtic	Brave, strong in conflict	
Brett	Old English, Celtic	A native of Brittany, Briton	Bret, Bretton
Briac	Celtic	Exalted	Brieg
Brian	Celtic	Strong	Bryan, Bryant, Briant, Briand

Caedmon	Celtic	Wise warrior	
Camlin	Celtic	Crooked line	
Carden	Celtic	From the black fortress	
Clancy	Celtic	Offspring of red-headed soldier	Clancey, Clan
Coalan	Celtic	Slender	Kayey
Cody	Celtic, Old English	Assistant, a cushion, possessions	Codie
Colin	Celtic, Greek	Youth, child, victor	Collin, Collins
Condon	Celtic	The dark-haired wise man	
Conner	Celtic	Desire, wise aid, wolf-lover	Conners, Connor, O'Conner, O'Connor, Conor, Conan
Corey	Celtic	Raven, from the hollow	Cory, Corry, Corrie, Correy
Craig	Celtic	From near the crag	Greg
Cullen	Celtic	Young animal, handsome	Culley, Cullin
Dermot	Celtic	Free of envy	Kermit
Derry	Celtic	Great lover, an ancient hero	
Desmond	Celtic, Latin	Man of the world, society	Desi, Des
Donnelly	Celtic	A brave black man	Donahue, Donnell, Donnel, Donner, Donovan, Donovon
Duane	Old English, Celtic	Dark, from the dunes	Dwayne, Dwane, Dwain, Dwaine, Duwayne, Wayne
Duff	Celtic	Dark faced, baker	Dough
Duncan	Celtic	Dark-skinned warrior	Dunc, Dun
Dunn	Celtic	Brown	Dunne
Edan	Celtic	Flame, fiery	
Egan	Gaelic, Celtic	Ardent, little fire	Egon, Egil

Evan	Celtic/Greek	Young warrior, well-born	Evans, Evanston
Farrell	Celtic, Old English	Courageous, man of valor	Farrel, Farrow
Fergus	Celtic	Of manly strength	Ferguson, Fergie, Fergy, Fergun
Ferguson	Celtic	Son of Fergus	
Ferris	Celtic, Latin	Rock, iron	Ferrys, Ferrell, Ferrel
Flynn	Celtic	Son of the red-haired man	Flinn, Flin, Flyn
Gallagher	Celtic	Eager aide	Gallagar, Gahan
Greg	Celtic	Fierce	
Irving	Celtic	Handsome, fair	
Kearney	Celtic	Warrior	
Keary	Celtic	Father's dark child	Kear, Care
Kegan	Celtic	Fiery	
Keir	Celtic	Dark-skinned	
Keith	Celtic; Welsh	Wood, wind; wood-dweller	
Kelvin	Celtic, Gaelic	Name of a river; from the narrow river	Kelvan, Kelven, Kelvyn, Kel
Kendr&eague;	Celtic	Loving male	Ken, Drea
Lorne	Celtic	Of Lorne	
Mannix	Celtic	Young monk	
Marmaduke	Celtic	Leader of the seas	Duke
Marvin	Celtic, Anglo-Saxon	Beautiful sea; good friend	Mervin, Mervyn, Merwin, Merwyn, Myrwyn, Murvyn, Myrvyn, Marv
Melvin	Celtic	Chief	Malvin, Melvyn, Mel, Mal

Merlin	Celtic, Anglo-Saxon, Welsh	Sea; falcon; sea hill	Merlyn, Marlin, Marlen, Marwin, Mervin, Merv, Merle
Monroe	Celtic, Scottish	Mouth of the Roe River; wheelwright	Munroe, Munro, Monro
Murray	Celtic	Sailor	Murry, Moray
Perth	Celtic	Thorny bush	
Ronan	Celtic	A pledge	
Scully	Celtic, Gaelic	Town crier	
Sean	Celtic	God's grace	Shawn, Shaun, Sian
Teague	Celtic, Gaelic	Poet	Tadhg
Tegan	Celtic	Doe	
Tiernan	Celtic, Gaelic	Lord	Tierney, Tyrnan
Tierney	Celtic	Lordly	
Torin	Celtic	Chief	
Torrance	Celtic, Gaelic	From the low hills	Torey, Torrey, Torry, Tori, Torr
Trevor	Celtic,	Cautious	Trefor
Urien	Celtic	Privileged birth	Turien, Turio
Vaughan	Celtic	Little, small	Vaughn
York	Old English, Celtic	Yew tree, from the farm of yew trees	Yorick

Chinese Male Baby Names

Name	Origin	Meaning	Similiar Names
Bo	Chinese	Great, vast	
Chen	Chinese, Korean	Gold; truth, treasure, pearl	
Jin	Chinese	Strength	
Lee	Chinese	Spiritual, deep-thinking	
Li	Chinese	Victory	
Shen	Chinese	Peach, symbol of long life	

Czech Male Baby Names

Name	Origin	Meaning	Similiar Names
Damek	Czech	Earth	
Evzen	Czech	Of noble birth	
Ladislav	Czech	Famous ruler	
Oldrich	Czech	One with riches and power	
Strom	German, Czech	Stream; tree	
Svaty Vavrinec	Czech	Saint Lawrence	
Vavrin	Czech	Laurel	
Vavrinec	Czech	Lawrence	
Zdenek	Czech	One from Sidon, a winding sheet	

Danish Male Baby Names

Name	Origin	Meaning	Similiar Names
Aksel	Danish	Peaceful Father	
Bardo	Danish	Son of the Earth	
Bendt	Danish	Blessed	Bent
Christer	Danish	Anointed, Follower of Christ	
Dagfinn	Danish	Day Finn	
Diederik	Danish	Ever Powerful ruler	
Eluf	Danish	Eternal Heir	
Erland	Danish	Stranger	Erlend
Flemming	Danish	Native of Flanders	
Frederik	Danish	Peaceful, Powerful ruler	Frederikke
Frode	Danish	Wisdom	
Gergers	Danish	Vigilant, Watchful	Greger
Hagen	Danish	Noble son	
Haldor	Danish	Rock, Thunder	Halldor, Halvor
Henning	Danish	Ruler of the home	
Jens	Danish	God is Gracious	
Jesper	Danish	Treasure	
Jokum	Danish	Founded by God	
Jorck	Danish	Farmer	Jorgn, Jorn
Kaj	Danish	Hen	
Karen	Danish	Blessed, Pure, Holy	
Keld	Danish	Sacrificial Kettle	Kjeld
Knud	Danish	Knot	
Kresten	Danish	Anointed	
Laurits	Danish	Crowned with Laurel	
Mads	Danish	Gift of God	
Mogens	Danish	Great	
Morten	Danish	Male	
Niels	Danish	Victorious people	
Olaf	Danish	Heir	Olav,Ole
Peder	Danish	Rock	
Poul	Danish	Small, Humble	
Preben	Danish	first battle	
Steen	Danish	Stone	

Thorbjorn	Danish	Thor's Bear	Thorstein, Torben, Torgeir, Torger, Torste
Tue	Danish	Thunder	
Tyge	Danish	Bullseye	

Dutch Male Baby Names

Name	Origin	Meaning	Similiar Names
Deman	Dutch	Man	
Killian	Gealic,Dutch	Fight, cell, strife; small water channel	Kilian, Kelian
Kyler	Dutch	Archer	
Maarten	Dutch	Fondness of war	
Roosevelt	Dutch	Field of roses	Rosey, Rosie
Wagner	Dutch	Wagon driver	

Egyptian Male Baby Names

Name	Origin	Meaning	Similiar Names
Amon	Celtic, Egyptian	The hidden	Ammon, Eamon, Eammon, Edmund
Moses	Hebrew, Egyptian, Greek	Saved; child; taken from water	Mose, Moe, Mosya, Moey, Moss, Moshe, Moishe, Mosheh, Moyes, Moyse
Paki	Egyptian	A witness	
Sabola	Egyptian	Prophet	
Zahur	Egyptian	A flower	

English Male Baby Names

Name	Origin	Meaning	Similiar Names
Abelard	Old German, Middle English	Resolute, keeper of the abbey larder	Abelardo, Eberhard
Ackley	Old English	Meadow of oaks	Ackerley
Acton	Old English	Town with many oaks	
Addison	Old English	Adam's son	Adison, Addisen
Aidan	Middle English, Gaelic	Help, little fire	
Ailen	Old English	Made of oak	
Aland	English	Bright as the sun	
Alcott	Old English	Old cottage	Alcot, Walcott, Walcot
Alden	Middle, Old English	Antique, old, wise protector, old friend	Aldan, Aldwin, Aldon
Alder	Middle, Old English	Birch tree, revered one	Elder, Aldus
Aldrich	Old English	Old king	Aldrych, Aldred, Aldren, Aldridge
Alfred	Old English	Wise counselor	Alf, Alfric, Alfie, Alfrid, Allie, Elfred, Fred, Freddie, Alfredo
Allard	Old English, Teutonic	Noble and brave	Alard
Alvin	Old English	Elf wine, noble friend	Alwyn
Amherst	English	Place name	
Amsden	Old English	From the ambroses valley	
Ansley	Old English	From the pastureland of the noble	

Atherol	Old English	Dweller at the spring farm	
Averill	Old English	Boar-warrior	Averil, Averell, Everill, Everil, Haverl, Haverhil
Bailey	French, English, Teutonic	Bailiff, fortification, able	Baily, Bayley, Bailee, Baylor
Ballard	Old English, French	A dancing song	
Bancroft	Old English	Bean field	
Barclay	Old English	Birch meadow	Barklay, Barkley, Barksdale, Berkeley, Berkley, Barks
Barden	Old English	Boar's den	
Barnett	Old English	Noble man	Barnet, Barret, Barrett, Barr
Baron	Old English	Noble man	Barron
Barse	English	Fresh-water perch	
Barton	English	From the barley farm	
Baul	English	Snail	
Bavol	English	Wind	
Beacher	Old English	Dweller by the beech tree	Beecher
Beaman	Old English	Beekeeper	Beeman
Beardsley	Old English	Beard, wood	
Bede	Old English	Prayer	
Beldon	Old English	Beautiful pasture, child of the unspoiled glen	Belden
Benson	English, Hebrew	Ben's son, excellent son	Bensen
Bentley	Old English	From the moor	
Bersh	English	One year	
Beval	English	Like the wind	
Birch	Old English	White	
Bishop	English	A bishop	
Blade	Old English	Glory	Bladen

Blaine	Gaelic, Old English	Thin, lean, source of a river	Blain, Blane
Blake	Old English	Fair-haired, pallid	Blakeley, Blachard, Blanco
Bob	Old English	Bright, famous	Róbert, Roberto, Rupert, Rubert, Robertson, Robin, Robinson, Robbins, Robben, Riobard, Robby, Robbie, Robey, Rober, Rab, Rob, Bobby, Robert, Bert, Berty, Tito, Dob, Dobbs
Bolton	Old English	Of the manor farm	
Bond	Old English	Tiller of the soil	
Booker	Old English	Beech tree	
Booth	Old English	Hut	Boothe
Borden	Old English, Old French	Near the boar's den, cottage	Bordan
Bowman	English	The archer	
Bradford	Old English	Broad crossing	
Bradley	Old English	Broad meadow	Braden, Brad, Brady, Braid, Bradney, Braeden, Braedon, Bradly
Bramwell	English	Place name	Branwell
Brandon	Old English	Fiery hill, sword	Branden, Brand, Bran, Brenden, Brendan, Brant, Brent, Brennen, Brennan, Branford
Bray	Old English	To cry out	
Brayden	Old English	Brave, broad	Brayton
Brennan	English	To brand	
Brent	Old English	Fiery hill, steep hill	Brentan
Brett	Old English, Celtic	A native of Brittany, Briton	Bret, Bretton
Brewster	Old English	Brewer	Brew

Brigham	Old English, Old French	One who lives near a bridge, soldier	
Brinley	Old English	Tawny	
Brishen	English	Born during a rain	
Brock	Old English	Badger	Braxton, Brocton
Broderick	Old English	Son of Roderick, from the broad ridge	Rick, Brod, Roderick
Bromley	Old English	Brush-covered meadow	Bromwell, Bromwood
Bronson	Old English	Son of Brown, son of the dark-skinned one	Bronwyn, Bronwen
Brown	Middle English	Colour	Broun, Bruno, Bruin, Bruins
Buckley	Old English	Meadow of deer	Buckminster, Buck, Bucky, Buckner
Bud	Old English, German	Herald, to puff up, friend	Buddy, Buddie, Budd
Burgess	Old English	Free citizen	Burg, Bergess, Bergen
Burle	Middle English	Knotted wood	Burl, Burleigh, Burley
Burne	Old English	Brook	Burns, Byrne, Burley
Burt	Old English	Fortress	Burton, Bert, Berton
Burton	English	Bright fame	
Calder	Old English	River of stones, stream	Caulder, Cal
Caldwell	Old English	Cold spring	Cadwell, Cadmus. Namesake
Calhoun	Old English	Warrior	
Carleton	Old English	Carl's town	Carlton, Charlton
Carlyle	Old English	Carl's island	Carlisle, Carl, Carlie, Carly, Lyle, Lisle
Carter	Old English	Cart driver	
Carver	Old English	Sculptor, wood carver	

Chad	Old English	Warlike	Chadwick
Chal	English	Boy, son	
Channing	Old English	Knowing	
Chapman	Old English	Merchant	
Charles	Old English	Manly, strong	Charlie, Charley, Charlton, Chuck, Chas, Chaz, Chip, Chuck, Carlos, Chico, Chick, Carlo
Chevalier	French, Old English	Knight, chase, hunt	Chevie, Chevy
Chilton	Old English	Farm by the spring	Chill, Chil, Chilly
Clark	Old English, French	Cleric, scholar	Clarke, Clarkson
Cleveland	Old English	Land near the hill, from the cliffs	Cleve, Clive, Cleavon
Clifford	Old English	Hill, near a slope	Cliff, Clifton
Clinton	Old English	Town near a hill	Clint
Cody	Celtic, Old English	Assistant, a cushion, possessions	Codie
Colby	Old English	Coal town	Kolby
Cole	Old English, Greek	Coal, victory of the people	Nicholas
Coleman	English	Charcoal burner, dove, peace	Colemann, Colman
Colton	Old English	Town of colt-breeding	Colston
Coty	English	Old house	
Courtland	Old English	The king's land, dweller in court	Cortland, Court, Cort
Creighton	Old English	Town near a creek	Creigh, Cree, Crichton
Crosby	English	Dweller near the town crossing	
Currier	Old English	Churn	Curran, Currie, Curry, Currey, Curren, Currer

Cynric	Old English	With royal might	
Dallin	Old English	Pride's people	
Dalton	Old English	Valley farm	
Damon	Greek, English	Constant, day	
Dane	Old English	From Denmark	
Danior	English	Born with teeth	
Darnell	English	Hidden nook	
Darrel	Old English	Beloved	Darryl, Darryll, Daryl, Daryll
Darren	Gaelic, Old English	Great, rocky hill	Darrin, Darin, Dare, Darryn
Darthmouth	English	Port's name	
Darwin	Old English	Beloved friend	Darwyn
Dayton	Old English	Bright town	Day, Daiton
Dean	Latin, Old English	Presiding official, valley	
Dempster	Old English	Judge	
Denver	Old English	Green valley	
Dickinson	Old English	Powerful, rich ruler	Dicken, Dickens, Dickenson, Dixon, Dix
Digby	Old English	Settlement near a ditch	
Dixie	Old English	Dick's son	Dixon, Dixi, Dixy
Donald	Old English	Ruler of the world, brown stranger	Donny, Don, Donnie, Donny, Donaldson, Donne, Donghal, Donal
Dorset	Old English	Tribe near the sea	Dorsey
Dover	Old English	Water	
Drake	Old English, Latin	Ale duck, dragon	
Duane	Old English, Celtic	Dark, from the dunes	Dwayne, Dwane, Dwain, Dwaine, Duwayne, Wayne
Dudley	Old English	People's meadow	Dud, Duddy, Dudly
Dugan	English	To be worthy	

Dunstan	Old English	From the brown rock quarry	
Durriken	English	Fortune-telling	
Durward	Old English	Gatekeeper	Durwood, Durwald, Durwin, Derwood
Dwennon	Old English	One of originality	Dwenn
Dwight	Old English	Fair, fair one	Dwyght, Dwighte, Dwyghte, Dwite, Dwyte, Doyt
Eaton	Old English	Riverside village	
Edgardo	Old English/French	Prosperous warrior	Edgar, Ed, Edgerton, Edger, Edgarton
Edison	English	Son of Edward	Edyson, Edson
Edmond	English	Prosperous protector	Edmund, Ed, Eddie, Ted, Teddy, Ede
Edward	Old English	Guardian of prosperity, guardian of the mists	Ed, Eddie, Eddy, Eduard, Edwardo, Eduardo, Edwards, Edwardson, Ted, Teddie, Ned, Neddie, Neddy, Edvard
Egerton	Old English	Edge	
Elden	Old English	Older	Elder, Alder, Eldred
Eldon	Old English	Ella's mound	
Eldridge	Old English	Old counselor	Elbridge
Elmar	Old English	Famous nobleman	Elmer, Elman, Elmore
Elton	Old English	From the old estate, Ella's town	Elten, Elroy
Emerson	Old English	Emery's son	Emersen, Emmerson, Emmyrson, Emyrson
Emmett	English	Hard worker, truth	Emmot, Emmott
Erskine	Gaelic/Old English	Dweller of the top of the cliff, green heights	

Esmond	Old English	Protective grace	Esmund, Desmond, Desmund
Ewing	Old English	Youth	Ewart
Fairfax	Old English	Blond-haired	Fairfield
Farley	Old English	Distant meadow	Fairley, Fairleigh, Farland, Fairly, Farly
Farrell	Celtic, Old English	Courageous, man of valor	Farrel, Farrow
Fenton	English	Marshland dweller	
Fielding	Old English	Field	Field, Fielder
Finlay	Scottish, English	Fair hero, sunbeam	Finn, Finnie, Finny, Finian, Finley, Fyn, Fynn, Finnian
Fleming	Old English	A native of Flanders	Flemming
Fletcher	Old English, Old French	Arrow maker	
Floyd	Old English	The hollow	
Forbes	Old English	Prosperous	
Ford	Old English	River crossing	
Forrester	English	Protector of the forest	
Free	Old English	In liberty	
Fuller	English	Clothing presser	
Fulton	Old English	Town near the field	
Gage	Old English, Old French	A pledge, a pawn	
Garfield	Old English	Promontory	Gar
Garrick	Old English	One who governs with a spear	
Garridan	English	You hid	
Gary	Old English, Latin, Teutonic	Spear carrier	Garry, Garrie, Garvey, Garvie, Garvin, Gervis, Gervais, Gervase, Garrick
Garyson	Old English	Son of Gary	Garrison, Garryson
Geoffrey	English	Heavenly place	Geoff

Germain	French, Middle English	From Germany; bud	German, Germain, Jarman, Jermyn, Jermain, Jermayne, Jermaine, Jermana
Gordon	English	From the cornered hill	
Granger	Old English	Farmer	
Grayson	Old English	Son of the bailiff	Gray
Gresham	English	From the grazeland	Grisham
Hadden	English	Child of the heather-filled valley	Haden
Hadley	Old English	Heath-covered meadow	
Halsey	Old English	From Hal's island	
Hamilton	Old English	Beautiful mountain	
Harden	Old English	From the Hare valley	
Harman	Old English	Soldier	
Harold	Old English	Army-power	
Harper	English	Harp player	
Harrison	English	Son of Harry	Harris
Hartley	English	From the deer pasture	
Harvey	Old English	Army warrior	Harv
Hayes	English	From the hedged place	Hazen
Hilton	Old English	Manor of the hill	
Holt	English	Son of the unspoiled forest	
Houston	English	Hill town	
Howard	English	Guardian of the home, watchman	Howe, Howie
Hugh	Old English	Bright in mind and spirit	Huey, Hugo
Hunter	Old English	Hunter	

Huntley	Old English	Hunter's meadow	
Jagger	Old English	A teamster	
Jal	English	Wanderer	
Jamison	English	Son of James	
Jarman	Old English	A German	
Jarvis	Old English	Driver, a conqueror	
Keane	English	Sharp, bold	Kean, Keen, Keene
Kell	English	From the spring	
Kemp	Middle English	Champion	Kempy, Kem, Kemper, Kemplen, Kempson
Kenelm	Old English	Brave helmet	
Kenley	Old English	Dweller at the king's meadow	Kenly
Kennard	English	Strong	
Kenneth	Gaelic, Scottish, Old English	Handsome; born of fire; royal oath	Ken, Kevin, Kennet, Kenny, Kenney, Kenn
Kenrich	Welsh, Old English	Chief hero; royal ruler	Kenrick, Kenway, Kenley, Kennard
Kent	Old English	Border, coast, bright white	
Kenton	Old English	From the king's estate	
Ker	English	House	
Keyon	Old English	Guiding, leading	Kieon, Key
King	Old English	Ruler	Kingsley, Kingston, Kingswell
Kinsey	Old English	Victorious prince	
Kipling	Middle English	One who cures salmon or herring	Kip
Kipp	Old English	Wearing a crown, sharply pointed hill	Kinnard, Kinnell, Kippy, Kipper

Knox	Old English	From the hills	Knoll
Ladd	Middle English	Young man	
Lander	Middle English, Greek	Property owner; lion man	Landor, Landry, Landis, Landers, Landman
Landon	Old English	Long hill	Landan, Landen
Lang	Old English, Old Norse	Long, tall	Langdon, Langford, Langley, Langston, Langhorne, Langtry
Latimer	Middle English	Interpreter	Lattimore
Lawson	Old English	Son of Lawrence	
Leland	Old English	From the meadow land	Leighton, Layton
Lensar	English	With his parents	
Lincoln	Old English	Home by the pond	Linc, Link
Lind	Old English	Linden tree	Lin, Linden, Lyndon, Lindell, Lindberg, Lindley, Lindon, Lindt, Linford, Linely, Linton
Linwood	Old English	Stream forest	
Litton	Old English	Hillside town	Lytton
Llewellyn	Old English	Ruling	
Lomar	Old English	Son of Omar	Omar
London	English	Fierce ruler of the world	
Lyman	Middle English	From the meadow	Leyman
Lyndon	Old English	Linden tree	Lindon, Linden
Lyre	Old English	A fork from river or glen	
Mac	Scottish, Irish, English	Son of	
Macon	Middle English	To make	Makon, Macomb
Macy	Old French, Old English	From Matthew's land; club	Macey, Mace, Maceo
Maitland	Old English	Dweller in the meadow	

Makepeace	Old English	Peace maker	
Mander	English	From me	
Manley	Old English	Man of the meadow	Manly, Manning, Mansfield, Manton, Manville, Manchester, Manheim
Manning	Old English	Son of the hero	Mann, Man
Marden	Old English	From the valley with the pool	
Marlow	Old English	From the hillside lake	Marlowe, Marlo
Marsden	Old English	Field near water	Marsdon, Marston, Marland, Marley, Marden, Marwood, Mardyth
Marshall	French, English	Keeper of the horses; steward	Marshal, Marschall, Marsh, Marshe
Mather	Old English	Strong army	
Maurice	French, Latin, Old English	Moorish; dark; moor land	Morris, Morse, Maury, Morry, Morey, Morrie, Moritz, Moriz, Morets, Meuriz, Moss, Morrell, Mauricio, Maurizio, Murray, Maryse, Morrison
Mavis	English	A small bird	Maves, Maeves, Maeve, Mauve, Meave, Maive
Maxwell	English	From the great well	
Mead	Old English	Meadow	Meade, Meed, Meid
Melor	English	Marx Engels Lenin October Revolution	
Melville	Anglo-Saxon, Old English	Hillside; town by the mill	Mel
Mendel	Hebrew, Middle English	Wisdom; repairer	Mel, Mendelssohn, Menachem, Menahem

Mercer	Middle English	Storekeeper	Merce
Merrick	English	Ruler of the sea	
Merrill	German, Old English	Famous; of the sea	Merral, Meril, Merrel, Meryl, Myrl, Myril, Merle, Merrick, Merton
Millard	Old English	Caretaker of the mill	
Miller	Old English	One who mills	Mills, Millson
Milton	Old English	From the mill town	Milten, Milty, Milt, Melton
Morley	English	Moor, meadow	Morlee, Morleigh, Morry, Morrie, Lee
Morven	Old English	Child of the sea	
Mull	Middle English	Grinder	Muller, Müller
Nash	Old English	Cliff	Nashe
Nelson	Old English	Son of a champion, son of Neil	Nealson, Neilson, Nilson, Nelly, Nellie
Nevin	Gaelic, Old English, German	Worshiper; middle; nephew	Nevins, Neven, Neffe
Newell	Old English, Old French	From the manor; kernel	Newall, Newlin, Newland, Newbold, Newgate, Newton
Newman	Old English	Newcomer	Neuman, Neumann, Numen, Newmie
Norman	Old French, Old English	Man from the north	Normie, Normal, Norm, Norris, Norville, Normand
North	Old English	From the north	Northcliff, Northrup, Norton, Norvin, Norwin, Norwyn, Norward, Norwell, Norwood, Nowles
Nyle	Old English	Island	
Oakes	English	From the oak-tree grove	
Oakley	Old English	From the oak meadow	
Ogden	Old English	From the oak valley	Oggie, Denny, Den
Olin	Old English	Holly	Olney, Olinda

Orman	Old English	Spearman	
Orson	Old English, Latin	Spearman's son; bear	Orsen, Orsin, Orsini, Sonny
Osbert	Old English	Inspired, divine	Osborn, Osborne, Osmar, Osmond, Osmund, Osted, Ostric, Osmen, Osman, Ossie
Osmond	Old English	God protector	
Oswald	Old English	Divinely powerful	Oswell, Ossie, Ozzie, Oswald, Oswall, Oswell, Oswaldo
Oswin	Old English	God friend	
Oxford	Old English	From where the oxen ford	Oxton, Oxon
Packard	Old English	One who packs	
Palmer	Old English	Palm bearing pilgrim	
Paris	English, Greek	City name; name of a God	
Parker	Old English	Cultivated land	Parke, Park, Parkley, Parks
Parr	Old English	From the stable	
Parry	Old English	Son of Harry	
Paxton	Teutonic, Old English	Trader; town of peace	
Pell	Old English	Scarf	Pelton, Pelham
Penley	Old English	Enclosed meadow	
Penn	Old English	Enclosure	
Perry	Middle English, Welsh	Pear tree; son of Harry	Pierrey, Parry, Perianne, Perian, Perrin, Perin
Pierce	Old English, Old French	Rock	Pearce, Piercy, Pears, Piers
Pierson	Old English	Son of Peter	Pearson
Prentice	Middle English	Apprentice	Prentiss

Preston	Old English	Dweller at the church, priest's settlement	Prescott, Presley, Priestley, Priestly, Priest
Putnam	Old English	From the sire's estate	Putney
Radcliff	Old English	Red cliff	Radcliffe, Radclyffe, Radclyf, Radford, Radley, Radnor, Rad
Rae	Old English	Doe	Ray, Rai
Raleigh	Old English	Dweller by the deer meadow	Rawley, Rawly, Rawls, Leigh, Lee
Ralph	Old English	Wolf, wise counselor	Ralf, Raff, Raffi, Rolf, Rolph, Raoul, Raul, Ralston
Ramsey	Old English	Ram's land	Ramsay, Ransden
Ransford	Old English	Raven's ford	
Ransley	Old English	Raven's meadow	
Ransom	Old English, Latin	Son of the shield; redeemer	Ransome, Ranson, Rankin, Rance
Raven	Old English	A raven	
Ravinger	Old English	Ravine	Ravi, Ravinia
Rawlins	Old English	Son of a little wise wolf	Rawlings, Rawson
Rayburn	Old English	From the deer stream	Rayfield, Rayford
Raymond	Old German, Old English	Worthy protector	Raymund, Ramon, Raimundo, Raimund, Reamonn, Rayner, Wray
Read	Old English	Red-haired, reed	Reed, Reid, Reading, Reade
Redford	Old English	From the red ford	Redfield, Redgrave, Redman, Redwald, Redd, Redding, Red
Reeve	Middle English	Bailiff	Reave, Reeves
Reginald	Old English	Powerful one	Reggie, Reggy, Reg, Reynolds, Reynold, Reinwald, Regnauld, Reinald, Renault, Rene, Rinaldo, Renato, Reinhold, Raghnall

Remington	Old English	From the raven's home	Remmy, Remy, Remmie, Remme
Rhodes	Middle English, Greek	Dweller by the crosses; roses	
Richard	Old German, Old English	Powerful ruler; brave one	Ricard, Ricardo, Richerd, Richman, Ricker, Richmond, Richardson, Rickward, Rickert, Rikkert, Rickard, Richart, Riocard, Ritchie, Rich, Rick, Rickie, Ricky, Rocco, Dick, Dickie, Dicky
Rider	Old English	Horseman	Ryder
Ridgley	English	By the meadow's edge	
Ridley	Old English	Reed clearing, cleared wood	
Rigby	Old English	Valley of the ruler	
Ripley	Old English	Dweller in the noisy meadow	Rypley, Rip
Rishley	Old English	From the wild meadow	Riston
Robert	Old English	Bright, famous	Róbert, Roberto, Rupert, Rubert, Robertson, Robin, Robinson, Robbins, Robben, Riobard, Robby, Robbie, Robey, Rober, Rab, Rob, Bobby, Bob, Bert, Berty, Tito, Dob, Dobbs
Rochester	Old English	Rock fortress	Rocky, Rock, Rocho, Roche, Rockley, Rockwell, Rockne, Rocker
Rodman	Old English	Famous	

Rodney	Old English	Famous one's island	Roddy, Rod
Roldan	English	Powerful, mighty	
Rowan	Gaelic, Old English	Red-haired; rugged	Rowen, Rowe, Rowell, Rowley, Rowson
Royce	English	Son of the king	
Rudd	English	Ruddy	Reed
Rudyard	Old English	From the red gate	Ruddy, Rudy
Russel	Old French, Old English	Red-haired; fox-like	Russel, Russ, Rusty, Rusti
Rutherford	Old English	From the cattle ford	Ruthren
Rylan	Old English	Dweller in the rye field	Ryland, Ryle, Rycroft, Ryman, Ryton
Sanders	Middle English	Alexander's son	Sander, Sandy, Sands, Sanderson, Saunders, Saunderson
Sandon	Old English	From the Sandy hill	
Sanford	Old English	Dweller at the sandy ford	Sanborn, Sandy, Sandford
Sawyer	Middle English	Woodsman	
Scott	Old English	From Scotland	Scot, Scotty, Scottie, Escott
Seabert	Old English	Sea-glorious	Seabright, Sebert, Seberg, Seabrook, Seabury, Sea
Seaton	Old French, Old English	From Baron's estate; sea town	Seeton, Seton, Seetin
Severin	English	River in England	
Seward	Old English	From the sea	Sewell, Severn
Seymour	Old French, Old English	Marshy land near the sea; taylor	Reminds me of Ingrid.
Shaw	Old English	A grove	
Sheldon	English	Protected hill	Shelton

Shelley	Old English	Clearing on a bank	Shelly, Shelli, Shell
Shepherd	Old English	One who heards sheep	Shepard, Sheppard, Shepley, Shep
Sherlock	Old English	White-haired	
Sherman	Old English	Wool cutter	Sherwin, Sherborne, Sherm
Sherwood	Old English	Bright forest	
Shipley	Old English	From the deep meadow	Shipton
Siddel	Old English	From the wide valley	Sydell, Sidwell
Skeet	Middle English	Speedy	Skeets, Skeat, Skeeter
Skye	English	Sky, sheltering	Sky
Slade	Old English	Child of the valley	
Smith	English	Blacksmith	Smyth, Smythe, Smitty, Smits
Snowden	Old English	From the snow-covered hill	Snowdun, Snow
Spalding	English	Divided field	Spaulding
Spencer	Old English	Dispenser, keeper	Spenser, Spence
Spike	Old English	Long, heavy nail	
Stanislaw	Polish, Old English	Camp glory; stone clearing	Stanislao, Stanislau, Stanislav, Stanislaus, Stanislav, Sztaniszláv, Stanislas, Stanislavsky, Stan, Aineislis, Stasio
Stanley	Old English	From the rocky meadow	Stanly, Stanleigh, Stanbury, Stanberry, Standish, Stanfield, Stanford, Stanhope, Stanmore, Stanton, Stanway, Stanwick, Stanwyck
Sterling	English	Genuine, valued	

Sterne	Middle English	Serious-minded	Stern, Stearn, Stearne
Stoke	English	Village	
Stokley	Old English	From the tree-stump meadow	Stockton, Stockwell, Stockman, Stokley
Stroud	Old English	From the thicket	Stroude, Stod
Studs	Old English	A house	
Sunny	English	Bright disposition, cheerful	Sunnie, Sunnee, Sonny, Sunday
Swain	Middle English	Knight's attendant	Swaine, Swayne, Swayze
Tab	Old German, Middle English	Briliant, drummer	Taber, Tabor, Tabbert, Taburer, Tabby
Tanner	Old English	Leather worker	
Tem	English	Country	
Tennyson	Middle English	Son of Dennis	Tennison, Tennessee, Tenny
Terrel	Old English	Thunderer	Terrill, Tirell, Terris, Tyrell, Rell
Thane	Old English	Attendant warrior	
Thatcher	Old English	Roof fixer	
Thorne	Old English	Thorn tree	Thorn, Thorndyke Thornton, Thornley
Thorpe	Old English	From the village	
Thurlow	Old English	From Thor	Thorald, Thorbert, Thorburn, Thorley, Thurmon, Thurman, Thurmond, Thurber, Thormond, Torold, Terrell
Todd	Middle English	Fox	Tod
Tomkin	Old English	Little Tom	Tompkin, Tomlin
Townsend	Old English	From the end of town	Towne, Townley, Townes
Tranter	Old English	Wagoner	
Tremayne	Old Cornish, English	House by the stones, farm with a stone monolith	Tremaine

Trent	Latin, Old English	Torrent, dweller by the Trent	Trenton
Trey	Middle English	Third born, three	Tray
Tripp	Old English	Traveller	
Truman	Old English	Disciple	Truesdale, True, Trueman
Tucker	Middle English	Tailor	Tuckman, Tuck
Turner	Middle English	Carpenter	
Twain	Middle English	Two pieces	
Tye	Old English	Enclosed	Tie, Tigh, Tighe, Tiegh, Tynan, Tai
Tyler	Middle English	Tiler, roofer	Tylor
Tyne	Old English	River	Tain, Tine
Ulrich	Old English, Old German	Wolf ruler	Ulric, Ulrick, Udolf, Ulger, Ull, Ulu
Upton	English	From the upper town	Upshaw
Vance	Middle English	Dweller at the windmill	
Wade	Middle English	A ford	Wadley, Wasdsorth
Wakefield	Old English	Wet field	Wake, Wakeley, Wakeman
Walker	Middle English	Cloth worker	
Wallace	Old English	Welshman	Wallis, Wallas, Wally, Wallie, Walsh, Welsh, Welch, Wallach
Walton	Old English	Dweller by the wall	Waller
Ward	Old English	To guard	Wardell, Warden, Wardley, Warfield, Warford, Warley, Warmond, Warton, Warwick
Warren	Old German, Middle English, Teutonic, French	Watchman, game keeper, enclosure, from La Varenne	Wareine, Warin, Warrener
Washington	Old English	From the estate of the wise one	

Watson	Old English	Son of Walter	Watkins, Watt
Waverly	Old English	From the tree-lined meadow	
Wayland	Old English	From the path land	Waylon, Way
Wayne	Old English	Wagon maker	Waggoner
Webster	Old English	Weaver	Weber, Webley, Webb
Welcome	English	Welcome guest	
Wells	Old English	From the springs	Welles, Weller, Welborne, Welby, Weldon, Welford, Welton
Wesley	Old English	West meadow	Wes, Wessely, Wess
Wetherby	Old English	Ram's meadow	
Wheaton	Old English	Wheat town	
Wheeler	Old English	A driver	
Whit	Old English	White	White, Whitey, Whitcomb, Whitby, Whitelaw, Whitfield, Whitford, Whitley, Whitlock, Whitman, Whitmore,Whittaker
Whitfield	Old English	From a small field	Whitley
Wilfred	Old English	Much peace	Wilfrid, Wilfried
Willow	English	Willow	
Wilmer	English	Will famous	
Winslow	Old English	From the friend's hill	Winchell, Windsor, Winfield, Winfred, Wingate, Winthrop, Winton, Wynton, Winward, Winfrey
Winston	Old English	Joy stone, victory town	
Winthrop	Old English	Friendly	
Wolf	English	Wolf	
Woodrow	Old English	Forester, row of houses by a wood	Woodruff, Woodward, Woodie, Woody

Wright	Old English	Craftsman, carpenter	
Wyatt	Old English, Old French	Little warrior, water	Wyeth
Wylie	Old English	Enchanting	Wiley
Wyndam	Old English	The field with the winding path	Windham, Wyn
Yale	German, Old English	One who pays or produces, corner of land	Yael
Yardley	English	Of the yard	
Yates	Middle English	Gate keeper	
York	Old English, Celtic	Yew tree, from the farm of yew trees	Yorick
Zane	Hebrew, Old English	God's grace, sea-friend	Zain

French Male Baby Names

Name	Origin	Meaning	Similiar Names
Aleron	French	Knight armor	
Algernon	Old French	Bearded	Algie
Ancel	Old German, French	Diety, servent, divine Helmt	Ansel, Ancell, Ancelot, Anselm, Anselme, Anselmo
Andrew	Greek, French	Manly, valiant, courageous	Anders, Andreas, Andres, Andre, Andrei, Andrey, Andries, Andros, Andy, Andie, Andrews, Drew, Andrea, Andrys
Armand	French	Of the army	Armond, Armande, Armando, Herman, Hermann, Arman
Audric	French	Old and wise rule	
Bailey	French, English, Teutonic	Bailiff, fortification, able	Baily, Bayley, Bailee, Baylor
Ballard	Old English, French	A dancing song	
Barry	French, Celtic, Welsh	Spear thrower, son of Harry, Marksman	Barrie, Barris, Barie, Barrymore
Bayard	Old French, Teutonic	Bay horse, red-brown hair	Baylor, Bayless, Baird
Beau	French	Handsome, beautiful	Beauregard, Bo
Beaumont	French	From the beautiful mountain	
Bellamy	Old French	Handsome friend	
Berenger	French	Courage of a bear	
Boden	Old French	Herald	

Bogart	French	Strong as a bow	
Boone	Latin, French	Good	Bono
Borden	Old English, Old French	Near the boar's den, cottage	Bordan
Boswell	Old French	Forested town	Bosworth, Bos
Boyce	French	Woodland	
Briand	French	Castle	
Brigham	Old English, Old French	One who lives near a bridge, soldier	
Bruce	French, Scottish	Thicket, woodlands	
Byron	French, Anglo-Saxon	From the cottage, bear	Byram, Byran
Cable	Old French	Rope	Cabel, Cab
Campbell	French	Beautiful field	Camp
Carel	French	Strong	
Case	Old French	Chest	
Chancellor	Old French	Secretary	Chance, Chauncey
Chandler	French	Candle maker	Chan, Chaney
Chaney	Old French	Oak-wood	
Chapin	Old French	Clergyman	
Chase	Old French	Hunter	
Cheney	Old French	From the oak forest	
Chevalier	French, Old English	Knight, chase, hunt	Chevie, Chevy
Ciel	French	From heaven	
Clark	Old English, French	Cleric, scholar	Clarke, Clarkson
Corbin	Old French	Raven, black hair	Corbett, Corbet, Corby, Corwin, Corwan, Corwyn
Curtis	Latin, Old French	Court, courteous	Curt, Curtys
Dartagnan	French	Leader	D'Artagnan
Delano	Old French	Of the night	
Desiderio	Latin, French	So long hoped for, crave, desire	Desi
Donatien	French, Latin	Gift	Donato

Edgardo	Old English/French	Prosperous warrior	Edgar, Ed, Edgerton, Edger, Edgarton
Egil	Norwegian, French	The edge or point, a sting	
Etienne	French	Estienne, Ettie, Etta	
Fletcher	Old English, Old French	Arrow maker	
Forest	Old French	Out of the woods	Forestt, Forrestt, Forster, Forrest
Foster	Old French	Forest keeper	
Francis	Latin, Old French	From France, free	Frank, Frankie, Franz, Franco, Ferenc, Franci
Franklin	Old French	Free man	Franklyn
Fraser	Old French	Strawberry	Frasier, Frazer, Fraiser, Frazier
Gage	Old English, Old French	A pledge, a pawn	
Gareth	Welsh, Norse, Old French	Gentle; enclosure; watchful	Garth, Garret, Garrett, Garreth, Gareth, Garit, Gary, Garry, Gar
Garland	Old French	Wreath	Garlan, Garlon, Garlyn, Gar
Gay	Old French	Merry	Gaye, Gae, Gai, Gaea
Gaylord	Old French	Brave strength	Gaylard, Gayelord
Germain	French, Middle English	From Germany; bud	German, Germain, Jarman, Jermyn, Jermain, Jermayne, Jermaine, Jermana
Granville	French	From the big town	
Guy	French, Teutonic	Guide; wood or wide	Gui
Hamlin	French	Little home-lover	
Jean	French	God is gracious	
Lance	Old French, Old German	Knight's attendant; land	Lancelot, Launcelot, Ancel
Leroy	Old French	The king	Leroi, Lee, Roy
Linus	Old French	Flaxen-haired	

Lionel	Old French	Young lion	Lyonel, Lionello, Lion, Lyon
Lyle	Old French	Island	Lisle, Lyell
Macy	Old French, Old English	From Matthew's land; club	Macey, Mace, Maceo
Marcel	French	Little hammer	Marcello, Marcellus, Marcellino
Marlon	Old French	Little hawk	Marlin, Marlyn, Marly, Marlo, Marlis, Marlys
Marshall	French, English	Keeper of the horses; steward	Marshal, Marschall, Marsh, Marshe
Maslin	Old French	Little twin	Maslen
Mason	French	Stoneworker	Masen, Mase
Maurice	French, Latin, Old English	Moorish; dark; moor land	Morris, Morse, Maury, Morry, Morey, Morrie, Moritz, Moriz, Morets, Meuriz, Moss, Morrell, Mauricio, Maurizio, Murray, Maryse, Morrison
Montgomery	French	Mountain hunter	
Mortimer	French	Still water	Morty, Mort
Neville	Old French	From the new farmland	Nevil, Nevile, Newland, Nev, Nevelson
Newell	Old English, Old French	From the manor; kernel	Newall, Newlin, Newland, Newbold, Newgate, Newton
Noel	French	Christmas	Noël, Nowell, Natale, Natal
Norman	Old French, Old English	Man from the north	Normie, Normal, Norm, Norris, Norville, Normand
Odil	French	Rich	
Oliver	Old Norse, Latin, Old French	Kind one; olive tree, peace	Olivier, Olivero, Olley, Olly, Ollie, Noll, Nolly

Orville	Old French	From the golden village	Orvalle, Orval
Page	French	Young attendant	Paige, Payge, Padgett
Pascal	French	Born at Easter	Paschal, Pasqual, Pasquale, Pascali, Pascha, Pace
Percival	Old French	Pierce the veil	Perceval, Percheval, Parsifal, Parsefal, Perce, Percy, Perci
Pierce	Old English, Old French	Rock	Pearce, Piercy, Pears, Piers
Porter	French	Gatekeeper, carrier	Porteur
Prewitt	Old French	Valiant one	Pruitt, Pruit, Prue
Quennel	Old French	Dweller by the oak tree	
Quincy	French	Estate belonging to Quintus	Quince, Quincey, Quin
Rance	French	A kind of Belgian marble	
Ranger	Old French	Dweller in the field	Rainger
Ray	French	Kingly	
Rivers	Latin, French	Stream of water	River, Rio
Roy	Old French, Gaelic	Regal one, red	Royal, Royale, Royall, Roi
Rush	French	Red-haired	Rousse, Rusk, Ruskin, Rust
Russel	Old French, Old English	Red-haired; fox-like	Russel, Russ, Rusty, Rusti
Sargent	Old French	Officer, to serve	Sargeant, Sergent, Sarge, Sergeant
Seaton	Old French, Old English	From Baron's estate; sea town	Seeton, Seton, Seetin
Seymour	Old French, Old English	Marshy land near the sea; Taylor	
Sinclair	French	Saint Clair	
Sinjon	French	Saint John	

Sumner	Old French	Summoner	Sumenor, Sumnor
Talbot	Old French	Reward	Tally, Tallie
Travis	Old French	Crossing	Travers, Trever
Troilus	French	Place name	
Tyson	Old French	Son of a German, son of Ty	
Vachel	French	Cow tender	
Valeray	Old French, Latin	Valor, strong	
Varden	Old French	From the green hill	Vartan
Vernon	French, Latin	Alder tree, springlike	Vern, Verda, Verne, Verney, Verna, Verneta, Vernia, Vernis, Virna, Vernal, Laverne, Lavinia
Warren	Old German, Middle English, Teutonic, French	Watchman, game keeper, enclosure, from La Varenne	Wareine, Warin, Warrener
Wyatt	Old English, Old French	Little warrior, water	Wyeth

Gaelic Male Baby Names

Name	Origin	Meaning	Similiar Names
Adair	Gaelic	Noble, exalted, oak-tree ford	Edgar
Aidan	Middle English, Gaelic	Help, little fire	
Alan	Gaelic, Celtic	Handsome, cheerful, noble	Allen, Allan, Alain, Alano
Angus	Gaelic, Celtic	Superb, unique	
Banning	Gaelic	Blond child	
Beacan	Celtic, Gaelic	Small, little one	Beagan
Blaine	Gaelic, Old English	Thin, lean, source of a river	Blain, Blane
Blair	Gaelic	From the plain, child of the fields	Blaire
Bowen	Gaelic	Son of Owen, yellow-haired	Bowie, Bo
Bram	Gaelic, Celtic	Raven	
Brendan	Gaelic	Little raven	
Brody	Gaelic	Ditch, unusual beard	
Brom	Gaelic	Raven	Bran, Bram
Cailan	Gaelic	Child	
Carlin	Gaelic	Little champion	
Carrick	Gaelic	Dweller on the rocky cape	
Cassidy	Gaelic	Clever	
Cavan	Gaelic	Handsome	
Cayden	Gaelic	Spirit of battle	
Corcoran	Gaelic	Of reddish complexion	
Curran	Gaelic	Hero	
Daley	Gaelic, Anglo-Saxon	Assembly, from the valley	Dailey, Daily
Daly	Gaelic	Advisor	
Darren	Gaelic, Old English	Great, rocky hill	Darrin, Darin, Dare, Darryn
Declan	Gaelic	Goodness	

Dempsey	Gaelic	Proud	
Devlin	Gaelic	Brave	
Dillon	Gaelic	Faithful	
Donovan	Gaelic	Dark warrior	
Doyle	Gaelic	Dark stranger	Doyl
Duglas	Gaelic	Dark stranger	
Egan	Gaelic, Celtic	Ardent, little fire	Egon, Egil
Erskine	Gaelic/Old English	Dweller of the top of the cliff, green heights	
Ewan	Gaelic	Well born	
Galen	Gaelic	Calm	
Gaynor	Gaelic	Son of the fair-haired one	
Glenn	Gaelic	Valley	
Grady	Gaelic	Noble, illustrious	
Iain	Gaelic	God's gracious gift	Ian
Keefe	Gaelic	Lovable and handsome, noble	Keefer, Keever
Keegan	Gaelic	Little fierce one	Keagan
Keeland	Gaelic	Little and slender	
Keenan	Gaelic	Little ancient one	Kienan, Keanan, Keen
Kelvin	Celtic, Gaelic	Name of a river; from the narrow river	Kelvan, Kelven, Kelvyn, Kel
Kendrick	Gaelic	Son of Henry	Kendric
Kennedy	Gaelic	Helmeted chief	Kennady, Kenny, Ken
Kenneth	Gaelic, Scottish, Old English	Handsome; born of fire; royal oath	Ken, Kevin, Kennet, Kenny, Kenney, Kenn
Kenyon	Gaelic	Blond-haired	
Kermit	Gaelic	Freeman	
Kern	Gaelic	Dark	
Kevin	Gaelic	Gentle, lovable	Kevan, Keven, Kev

Kieran	Gaelic	Small and dark-skinned	Kiernan, Kieron, Key, Kerwin, Kirwin, Kerry, Kern, Kerr, Ceirnin, Carra, Ciaran
Killian	Gaelic, Dutch	Fight, cell, strife; small water channel	Kilian, Kelian
Kinnel	Gaelic	Dweller at the head of the cliff	
Kyle	Gaelic	Handsome, near the chapel, narrow, narrow channel, strait	Kylie, Kyleigh, Leigh, Lei, Kyli
Lawler	Gaelic	Softspoken	
Lennon	Gaelic	Cloak, little cape	Lenin
Lon	Gaelic	Fierce	Lonny
Mackenzie	Gaelic	Son of the wise leader	Mackie, Kenzie, Max, Mackenzy
Murphy	Gaelic	Sea warrior	Murphee, Murphree
Neal	Gaelic	Champion	Neil, Neill, Nial, Niall, Neale, Neel, Niels, Niel, Niles, Nels, Nils, O'Neill, Neely
Nevin	Gaelic, Old English, German	Worshiper; middle; nephew	Nevins, Neven, Neffe
Nolan	Gaelic	Noble	Nolen, Nolin, Nolyn, Nowlan
Oran	Gaelic, Hebrew	Pale one; pine	Orin, Orren, Oren, Orran, Orrin, Oram, Orrie

Oren	Hebrew, Gaelic	Ash-tree, pale; pine tree	
Parlan	Gaelic	Ploughman, farmer	
Phelan	Gaelic	Little wolf	
Quillan	Gaelic	Club	
Regan	Gaelic	Little king	Reagan, Rayghun, Reagen, Regen, Regino, Regent
Renny	Gaelic	Small but mighty	
Riordan	Gaelic	Poet	Reardon
Roarke	Gaelic	Famous ruler	Ruark, Rourke, Rorke
Rooney	Gaelic	Red-haired	Roon, Roone, Rune
Rory	Gaelic	Red king	Rurik, Roric, Ruaidhri
Rowan	Gaelic, Old English	Red-haired; rugged	Rowen, Rowe, Rowell, Rowley, Rowson
Roy	Old French, Gaelic	Regal one, red	Royal, Royale, Royall, Roi
Scully	Celtic, Gaelic	Town crier	
Sheehan	Gaelic	Little peaceful one	Sheen
Slevin	Gaelic	Mountaineer	
Sloan	Gaelic	Warrior	Sloane, Slone
Sullivan	Gaelic	Black eyes	Sullyvan
Sully	Gaelic	To stain	
Sweeny	Gaelic	Little hero	Sweeney
Teague	Celtic, Gaelic	Poet	Tadhg
Tiernan	Celtic, Gaelic	Lord	Tierney, Tyrnan
Torrance	Celtic, Gaelic	From the low hills	Torey, Torrey, Torry, Tori, Torr
Trevor	Celtic, Gaelic	Cautious	Trefor

German Male Baby Names

Name	Origin	Meaning	Similiar Names
Abelard	Old German, Middle English	Resolute, keeper of the abbey larder	Abelardo, Eberhard
Adalgiso	Old German	Noble hostage	Adelchi
Adalrico	Latin, Old German	Noble, powerful and rich	Adalricus, Adalrich
Adelbert	Old German	Famous for nobility	Adalberto, Adalbert, Bertl, Bert, Adi, Adelberto
Adelfried	Old German	Who protects the descendants	Adalfrid, Adelfrid, Adalfredo, Adalfreddo
Adelino	Old German	Noble	
Adelmo	Old German	Noble protector	Adalhelm, Adelhelm
Ademaro	Old German	Glorious in battle	Hadumar, Adimaro
Adler	German	Eagle	
Adolph	German	Noble wolf, noble hero	Adolf, Adolphe, Adolphus, Adolfus, Adolpho, Adolfo, Adaulfo
Ahren	Old German	Eagle	
Alaric	Old German	Noble ruler	
Albert	German	Noble and bright	Alberto, Albertus, Albrecht, Adelbert, Aubert, Elbert, Bertel, Berty, Bertie, Al, Alby, Albie
Aldous	Old German	Old wealthy	Aldus, Aldo

Alger	Old German	Noble warrior	Elgar, Elger
Alphonse	Old German	Noble estate, eager	Alfonse, Alfons, Alphonso, Alonso, Alonzo, Alonza, Alfonso
Ancel	Old German, French	Diety, servent, divine Helmt	Ansel, Ancell, Ancelot, Anselm, Anselme, Anselmo
Arnold	German	Eagle, powerful	Arnaud, Arnault, Arnie, Arnald, Arno, Arne, Arnell, Arnel, Arness, Arnot, Arnaldo
Baldwin	German	Bold friend	Baldwyn, Maldwyn, Baldovino, Balwin
Barend	Germanic	Bear	
Bergen	German	Mountain dweller	Bergan, Bergin
Bernard	German	Bold as a bear	Barnard, Barney, Barnie, Bernd, Berndt, Bern, Berne, Bernardo, Bernhard, Bernhardt, Bernie
Bertram	German	Bright	Bertrem, Bertil, Bertol, Bert
Bingham	German	Kettle-shaped hollow	Bing, Binghamton, Binghampton, Bin
Blaz	Old German	Unwavering protector	Blaze
Brandeis	German	Dweller on a burned clearing	

Bud	Old English, German	Herald, to puff up, friend	Buddy, Buddie, Budd
Burke	German	Birch tree	Bourke, Burk, Birk, Birke
Conrad	Old German	Brave counselor	Connie, Rad, Konrad, Kon, Con, Conroy, Cort, Corrado
Cort	Old German	Bold	Kurt, Curt, Kurtis, Curtis
Dagobert	German	Shining sun	
Derek	Old German	Ruler	Derik, Dirk, Derick, Derrick, Derrik, Derych, Derry, Der, Derex
Dieter	German	The people's ruler	
Dutch	German	The German	
Eberhard	Germanic	Strong wild boar	Everett, Everet, Everard, Eberhart, Eberardo
Edwin	German	Prosperous friend, heir's axe	Edwyn
Egbert	German	Sword, famous, shiny	
Egmont	German	Weapon, defender	
Eldwin	Old German	Old friend	
Ellery	German/Latin	One who lives near the elder tree, cheerful	Elery, Ellory, Elory, Ellary, Elary
Emery	German	Ruler of work, powerful home	Emory, Emmery, Emmory
Emil	Old German	Industrious, to emulate	
Ernest	Old German	Earnest, vigorous	Ernie, Erni, Erny, Ernst, Earnest, Ernesto
Ferdinand	Old German	Courageous traveler	Ferdie, Ferdy, Ferde, Ferd, Fernando, Fernandas

Frederick	Old German	Peaceful ruler	Frederic, Fred, Freddie, Freddy, Fritz, Fritzie, Fritzi
Fremont	Old German	Guardian of freedom	
Garin	Old German	Warrior	
Geert	Germanic	Brave strength	
Gerard	Old German	Spear-brave	
Hackett	German	Little woodsman	
Hahn	German	Rooster	
Hank	German	Ruler of an estate	
Hastings	German	Swift one	
Heller	Old German	The sun	
Helmuth	German	Helmet, protector, courage	Helmuth, Heli
Henry	Old German	Ruler of the home	Henri, Henrik
Herman	Old German	Man of the army	Harman
Imre	German	Great king	
Johann	German	God's gracious gift	Janez
Kasch	German	Like a blackbird	
Kay	Old Welsh, Old German	Rejoicer; fort	Kay, Kai, MacKay
Kellen	German	Wwamp	
Kiefer	German	Barrel-maker	
Lance	Old French, Old German	Knight's attendant; land	Lancelot, Launcelot, Ancel
Lear	German	Of the meadow	
Leonard	Old German	Lion-hearted	Lennard, Lenard, Lennart, Leonardo, Leonhard, Leon, Leo, Lennie, Lenny, Len, Lénárd, Leonárd, Leó
Leopold	Old German	Bold leader	Luitpold, Leupold, Leopoldo

Louis	Old German	Famed warrior	Lewis, Lewes, Luis, Louie, Lewie, Lou, Lew, Lu, Ludwig, Ludvig, Luigi, Lodovico, Luthias, Llewellyn, Clovis, Chlodwig, Lajos
Luther	Old German	Warrior	Lutera, Lothaire, Lotario
Manfred	Old German	Man of peace	Manny, Fred
Mayer	German, Latin, Hebrew	Farmer; greater; bringer of light	Meyer, Meir, Meier, Mayr, Myer, Mayor, Myerson
Merrill	German, Old English	Famous; of the sea	Merral, Meril, Merrel, Meryl, Myrl, Myril, Merle, Merrick, Merton
Meyer	German	A farmer	
Miles	Latin, Old German, Greek	Soldier; merciful; millstone	Myles, Milo, Milos, Milan, Milah, Miles, Mila
Nevin	Gaelic, Old English, German	Worshiper; middle; nephew	Nevins, Neven, Neffe
Norbert	Old German	Blond hero	
Odell	Old German, Greek, Danish	Little wealthy one; ode; otter	Ode, Odie, Odis
Omar	Arabic, Hebrew, German	First son, disciple; gifted speaker; famous	Omer
Otis	Greek, Old German	Acute; wealthy	Otto, Odo, Otho, Othello, Otello, Otilio
Penrod	Old German	Esteemed commander	Penn

Raymond	Old German, Old English	Worthy protector	Raymund, Ramon, Raimundo, Raimund, Reamonn, Rayner, Wray
Raynard	Old German, Old Norse	Brave one; mighty army	Raynard, Renard, Reinhard, Raynor, Reinhart, Rinehart, Renaud, Reynaud, Reynart, Reyner, Rey
Redmond	Old German	Adviser	
Richard	Old German, Old English	Powerful ruler; brave one	Ricard, Ricardo, Richerd, Richman, Ricker, Richmond, Richardson, Rickward, Rickert, Rikkert, Rickard, Richart, Riocard, Ritchie, Rich, Rick, Rickie, Ricky, Rocco, Dick, Dickie, Dicky
Ring	Old German	A ring	Ringling, Ringo
Ritter	Old German	Knight	Ritt
Roderick	Old German	Famous one	Rodrick, Broderick, Rodrigo, Roderich, Rodrigue, Rodney, Rod, Rodd, Roddy, Rodman, Rodmond, Rory, Rick, Ricky

Roger	Old German	Famous spearman, quiet	Rodger, Rodgers, Rogers, Rogerio, Rog, Ruggiero, Rudiger, Rodiger, Rutger, Rüdiger
Roland	Old German	From the famous land	Rolland, Rowland, Rollan, Rollin, Rollins, Rolando, Rodhlann, Rowe, Rollo, Rolly, Orlando, Rolt, Roland
Roth	German	Red-haired	
Rudolph	Old German	Wolf	Rudolf, Rodolf, Rodolphe, Rodolfo, Raoul, Rudy, Rudie, Rudi, Rolf, Rolph, Rollo, Rollin, Dolph
Stein	German	Stone	Steyn, Stine, Styne, Steiner, Steen, Steinway, Steinbeck, Steinberg, Steinmetz
Strom	German, Czech	Stream; tree	
Tab	Old German, Middle English	Briliant, drummer	Taber, Tabor, Tabbert, Taburer, Tabby

Theobold	Old German	The boldest	Teoboldo, Tibalt, Tybalt, Thebault, Thibaud, Thibaut, Theo
Ulrich	Old English, Old German	Wolf ruler	Ulric, Ulrick, Udolf, Ulger, Ull, Ulu
Vid	German	Sylvan man	Vida, Vidos
Walter	Old German	Powerful warrior, rule amry	Walt, Wally, Walther, Watson, Watkins, Gautier, Gauthier, Ualtar
Warner	Old German	Defending army	Werner
Warren	Old German, Middle English, Teutonic, French	Watchman, game keeper, enclosure, from La Varenne	Wareine, Warin, Warrener
Yale	German, Old English	One who pays or produces, corner of land	Yael
Zelig	Old German	The blessed one	

Ghanese Male Baby Names

Name	*Origin*	*Meaning*	*Similiar Names*
Adeben	Ghanese	Twelfth-born son	
Ashon	Ghanese	Seventh-born son	
Kontar	Ghanese	Only child	
Tano	Ghanese	Name of river	

Greek Male Baby Names

Name	Origin	Meaning	Similiar Names
Achilles	Greek	Without lips, brown, dark	Achille, Achill, Achilla, Akilleys, Aquila, Achilleo
Adelphos	Greek	Brother	Aldelfo, Adelfio
Adonis	Greek	Man loved by Aphrodite, handsome	Adone
Adrastos	Greek	Undaunted	Adrasto
Adrian	Greek, Latin	Rich, wealthy, dark one	Adrien, Adrie, Hadrian, Adrianus, Adriano, Hadrianus
Aeneas	Greek	Worthy of praise	
Aetos	Greek	Eagle	
Agatone	Greek	Good, kind	
Alcander	Greek	Strong	Alcindor, Alcandor
Alexander	Greek	protector of mankind	Alec, Alek, Aleks, Alecks, Aleksy, Alex, Alesandro, Aleksandr, Alessandro, Alejo, Alexei, Alysander, Alexandre, Alejandro, Aleksander, Alastair, Iksander, Sandro, Sander, Sanders, Sandor, Xander
Amarus	Greek	Unfading love	

Ambrose	Greek	Immortal	Ambrosia
Anatole	Greek	From the East	Anatoly
Andreus	Greek	Son of river Peneius	
Andrew	Greek, French	Manly, valiant, courageous	Anders, Andreas, Andres, Andre, Andrei, Andrey, Andries, Andros, Andy, Andie, Andrews, Drew, Andrea, Andrys
Angelo	Greek	Heavenly messenger	Angelico
Anieli	Greek	Manly	
Anker	Greek	Manly	
Anthony	Latin, Greek	Priceless, flourishing, flower	Anthoney, Antonius, Anton, Antony, Antonio, Tony, Toni, Tonio, Tonie, Tone, Tee, Toney, Antonio, Anthony, Antone, Antoine, Anth, Nee
Ares	Greek	God of war	
Argus	Greek	Bright, watchful	
Arion	Greek	Musician	
Aristo	Greek	Best	
Arsen	Greek	Strong	
Arsenio	Greek	Manly, virile	
Artemis	Greek	Moon	Artemus, Artie
Athan	Greek	Immortal	
Attis	Greek	Handsome boy	Attisian, Attisa

Basil	Greek, Arabic	Royal, brave	Basile, Basilo, Basilia, Basia, Vasilis, Vasily
Bastiaan	Greek	Venerable	Bastian
Belen	Greek	An arrow	
Bemus	Greek	Platform	
Calisto	Greek	Most beautiful	Cal, Kalisto, Kal
Christian	Greek	Anointed, follows Christ	Christiaan, Kristian, Chris, Chrestian, Karston, Karstan,
Christopher	Greek	Christ-bearer	Kristofer, Kristopher, Christof, Kristof, Chris, Kris, Kit, Christophe, Kester, Cristobel, Cristoforo
Christos	Greek	Christ	Christo, Cristo, Kristo
Cole	Old English, Greek	Coal, victory of the people	Nicholas
Colin	Celtic, Greek	Youth, child, victor	Collin, Collins
Corban	Greek	A gift devoted to God	Qorbin, Korban
Cosmo	Greek	Order, universe	Comsy, Kosmos
Cyrano	Greek	From Cyrene	Siranno, Sirano, Cirano, Syrano, Syranno
Cyril	Greek	Lordly, proud	Cyra, Kyril, Cirillo, Cy
Damen	Greek	Taming	

Damian	Greek	Tamer, divine power, fate	Damien, Damon, Daimen
Damon	Greek, English	Constant, day	
Deacon	Greek	Servent, messenger	Declan
Demetrius	Greek	Lover of the earth, given to the Earth goddess	Demitiri, Dimitri, Dimitry, Dimity, Dmitry, Dmitri, Demeter
Denes	Greek, Hungarian	Wine, drama	
Dennis	Greek	Of Dionysus	Denis, Dennys, Dennison, Denniston, Denzel, Denzil, Denzell, Denit, Dennit, Dion, Denny, Tennis, Tennyson, Dionysus
Deo	Greek	Godlike	
Dorian	Greek	Place name	Dorien, Dorie, Dorrien, Dorrian, Dory
Dymas	Greek	Father of Hecate	
Eryx	Greek	Son of Aphrodite and Poseidon	
Eudor	Greek	Good gift	Dora
Eugene	Greek	Born lucky	Gene,
Eugenia	Greek	Born lucky	Eugenie
Eustace	Greek	Fruitful	Stace, Stacie
Evan	Celtic/Greek	Young warrior, well-born	Evans, Evanston
Evander	Greek	Early founder of rome, benevolent ruler	

George	Greek	Farmer, to work the earth	Georg, Georges, Georgio, Giorgio, Giorgis, Georgius, Georgie, Georgi, Georgy, Geordie, Goran, Jorge, Jorges, Jorgen, Jerzy, Jiri, Juro, Jurik, Jur, Jeorg, Jürgen, Jurgen, Jurek, Jorrin, Jurgi, Yegor, Yura, Yurchik, Yurik, Yusha, Yurko, Yoyi, Yuri, Egor, Zhorka, Seiorse
Homer	Greek	Promise	
Jason	Greek	Healer	
Karsten	Greek	Blessed, anointed one	
Kozma	Greek	Decoration	
Krischnan	Greek	Christian	Krister
Lander	Middle English, Greek	Property owner; lion man	Landor, Landry, Landis, Landers, Landman
Leander	Greek	Lion man	Liander, Leandre, Leandro
Leonidas	Greek	One who is bold as a lion	Leonidis, Leonid
Lysander	Greek	Liberator, emancipation	
Lysandra	Greek	Liberator, emancipation	
Melancton	Greek	Black flower	Melanchthon

Miles	Latin, Old German, Greek	Soldier; merciful; millstone	Myles, Milo, Milos, Milan, Milah, Miles, Mila
Moses	Hebrew, Egyptian, Greek	Saved; child; taken from water	Mose, Moe, Mosya, Moey, Moss, Moshe, Moishe, Mosheh, Moyes, Moyse
Myles	Greek	Inventor of the corn mill	
Myron	Greek	Sweet oil	
Napoleon	Greek, Italian	Lion of the woods; from the city of Naples	Nappie, Nappy, Nap, Leon, Leo
Narcissus	Greek	Self-love	Narcisus
Neo	Greek	New	
Nestor	Greek	Traveler, wisdom	Nesta, Nest
Nicholas	Greek	Victorious people	Nicolas, Nikolas, Nikolie, Niko, Nikolaus, Nicklaus, Nicola, Nick, Nicky, Nikki, Nikita, Nickita, Nikos, Nikolai, Nikola, Nicholai, Nicanor, Nikos, Nicos, Nichol, Nichols, Nicolson, Nicol, Nicolo, Nikolos, Nicko, Nicodemus, Nils, Niles, Nixon, Cole, Colin, Colet, Claus, Klaus, Klas, Klaas, Miklós
Nicodemus	Greek	Victory of the people	

Obelix	Greek	Pillar of strength	Obelius
Odell	Old German, Greek, Danish	Little wealthy one; ode; otter	Ode, Odie, Odis
Odysseus	Greek	Full of wrath	
Orion	Latin, Greek	Dawn, east; son of fire, the hunter	Orien, Oris
Orrin	Greek	Mountain	Orestes, Orest
Otis	Greek, Old German	Acute; wealthy	Otto, Odo, Otho, Othello, Otello, Otilio
Owen	Old Welsh, Greek	Warrior; well born	Owyn, Ewan, Ewen, Owens
Panos	Greek	A rock	
Panthea	Greek	Of all the Gods	
Paris	English, Greek	City name; name of a God	
Peder	Greek	Stone	
Philip	Greek	Horse lover	Phillip, Philipe, Philippos, Philo, Phillips, Phelps, Phipps, Philipson, Phillips, Philby, Phil, Philly, Felipe, Filippo, Filip, Filbert
Phoenix	Greek	Mystical bird, purple	
Platon	Greek	Broad-shouldered	
Rhodes	Middle English, Greek	Dweller by the crosses; roses	
Sofronio	Greek	Self-controlled	Sophronio
Soterios	Greek	Saviour	

Stephen	Greek	Crown	Steven, Stefan, Stephan, Stepan, Steve, Stevie, Steven, Stefano, Stephens, Stevens, Stevenson, Stephenson, Etienne, Esteban, Estevan, Steffan
Talos	Greek	Giant protector of Minos island	
Tarasios	Greek	Of Tarentum	Taras
Thanos	Greek	Noble	
Theodore	Greek	Gift of God	Theodor, Teodore, Teodoro, Teddy, Ted, Feodor, Fedor, Fyodor, Telly, Teodor
Theophilus	Greek	Beloved of God	
Theron	Greek	Hunter	
Thomas	Greek	Twin	Tomas, Tomaso, Tom, Thom, Thos, Tommy, Thompson, Thomson, Massey, Tamas
Tibalt	Greek	People's prince	
Timeus	Greek	Perfect	
Timoleon	Greek	I honor what I say	
Timon	Greek	Worthy	
Timothy	Greek	Honoring God	Timotheus, Timoteo, , Timmy, Timmie, Tim, Timon, Timo,

Titus	Greek	Of the giants	Tito, Titan
Tymon	Greek	Honoring God	
Tyrone	Greek	King	Tyron
Vasilios	Greek	With royal blood, regal	Vasily, Wasily, Vassily
Xanthus	Greek	Yellow	
Xenos	Greek	Stranger	
Zarek	Greek	May God protect the king	
Zefirino	Greek	Wind of spring	Zefferino, Zefiro
Zeno	Greek	Of Zeus	
Zenobio	Greek	Strength of Jupiter	
Zenos	Greek	Gift of Zeus	Zen
Zephyr	Greek	Wind	Zephirin
Zero	Greek	Seeds	
Zeth	Greek	Investigator, researcher	Zeticus, Zetico
Zoello	Greek	Son of Zoe	Zoellus
Zoilo	Greek	Lively	

Hawaiian Male Baby Names

Name	Origin	Meaning	Similiar Names
Bane	Hawaiian	Long-awaited child	
Kahoku	Hawaiian	Star	
Kale	Hawaiian	Strong and manly	
Keona	Hawaiian	God's gracious gift	Keowynn
Leilani	Hawaiian	Heavenly flower, heavenly child	
Meka	Hawaiian	Eyes	

Hebrew Male Baby Names

Name	Origin	Meaning	Similiar Names
Aaron	Hebrew, Arabic	Shining light, high mountain, messenger	Aron, Ahron, Arron
Abbott	Arabic, Aramaic, Hebrew	Father	Abbot, Abba, Abbe, Absa
Abdiel	Hebrew	Servent of God	Abdia
Abel	Hebrew, Assyrian	Breath, child	Able, Abell, Abele, Ibila
Abijah	Hebrew	The Lord is my Father	Abia, Abbiah, Abiam
Abner	Hebrew	Father of light	
Abraham	Hebrew	Father of a multitude	Abram, Avraham, Avram, Avrom, Abe, Abie, Abra, Ibrahim, Braham, Bram, Abramo, Abran, Abramio
Abrasha	Hebrew	Father	
Acacio	Hebrew	The Lord holds	Achazio
Adam	Hebrew	Earth, created by God	Adams, Adamson, Adie, Addie, Addy, Adan, Adem, Adamo, Adamah
Addai	Hebrew	Man of god	
Addo	Teutonic, Hebrew	Happy, ornament	Adah, Ado
Adlai	Hebrew	My witness, refuge of God	
Adley	Hebrew	Just	
Admon	Hebrew	Red peony	
Adon	Hebrew	Lord	Adone

Ahab	Hebrew	Uncle	
Ahmik	Hebrew	Strength of God's flock	
Aitan	Hebrew, African	Fights of possession	
Amiel	Hebrew	God of my people	
Amos	Hebrew	Troubled	
Ardon	Hebrew	Bronze	
Ari	Hebrew	Lion	Aree
Armon	Hebrew	Castle	
Arnon	Hebrew	Rushing stream	
Asher	Hebrew	Fortunate, lucky, blessed, happy	Asser, Ashe, Ashbel, Anschel
Axel	Hebrew, Swedish	Divine reward; divine source of life	Axtel
Barabas	Hebrew	Barabba	
Barnabas	Hebrew	Son of prophecy	Barnaby, Barney, Barnie, Barn
Bartholomew	Hebrew	Furrow, hill	Barth, Bart, Barthol, Bartel, Bartlett, Bartley, Barton, Bertol, Bartold, Bat, Bart, Tholy, Tolly, Bartolomeo, Parlan
Baruch	Hebrew	Blessed	
Benjamin	Hebrew	Son of my right hand	Benji, Benjie, Bennie, Benny, Ben, Beniamino
Benson	English, Hebrew	Ben's son, excellent son	Bensen
Beryl	Hebrew	Dazzling jewel	Bijou
Brighton	Hebrew	The one who is loved	Bright, Brie
Britt	Hebrew	The helpful one	
Cain	Hebrew	Craftsman	Kain, Caino, Caine
Chaika	Hebrew	Life	

Chaim	Hebrew	Life	Cahyim, Cahyyam, Haim, Haym, Cahya
Dagan	Hebrew	Grain or corn	
Daniel	Hebrew	My judge is the Lord	Danny, Daniele, Danielus, Dan, Danni, Daniels, Danilo, Danil
David	Hebrew	Beloved one	Dave, Davey, Davy, Davie, Davi, Davyd, Davis, Davidson, Dawes, Dawson, Dewi, Dewey, Devlin, Dabney
Doron	Hebrew	Gift	
Dov	Hebrew	Bear	
Eban	Hebrew	Stone	Ebenezer, Eben
Eisig	Hebrew	He who laughs	
Eli	Hebrew	Elevation	
Elijah	Hebrew	Jehovah is God	Elias, Ellis, Eliha, Elyas, Ellison, Ellsworth, Ellys, Ilya, Ilja, Eliakim, Elia, Eli
Eliot	Hebrew	Hight	Eli, Ely, Elliot, Elliott, Eliott
Elkan	Hebrew	Ge belongs to God	
Emanuel	Hebrew	God is with us	Emmanuel, Emmanuel, Immanuel, Imanuel, Manuel, Manny
Ephraim	Hebrew	Very fruitful	Efrem, Ephrem

Ethan	Hebrew/Latin	Strong, firm, constant	Ethen, Etan
Ethel	Hebrew	Noble	Adele, Ethelred, Ethelbert
Ezekiel	Hebrew	Strength of God	Ezekyel
Ezio	Hebrew	Friend, lover	Azio
Ezra	Hebrew	Helper, salvation	Ezer, Ezri, Ezzret
Gabai	Hebrew	Delight, adornment	
Gabriel	Hebrew	God is my strength	Gabe, Gabino, Gabryel, Gabriello, Gavrila, Gabby, Gab, Gable
Gideon	Hebrew	Mighty warrior	Giddy, Gid
Isaac	Hebrew	Laughing one	
Isaac	Hebrew	He will laugh	Ike
Isaiah	Hebrew	Salvation of the Lord	
Israel	Hebrew	Prince of God, may God reign	
Itzak	Hebrew	Laughter	Jitzak
Jacob	Hebrew	Held by the heel	Jacques, Jake, Jeb, Jock, Jacobe, Iacob, Iacobe, Jakob
James	Hebrew	Supplanter	Seamus, Jaime, Jamie, Jim, Jimmy
Jared	Hebrew	One who rules	Jarett, Jarrett
Jarlath	Hebrew	A tributary lord	
Jaron	Hebrew	To cry out, singing	Yaron
Jedidiah	Hebrew	Beloved of the Lord	
Jeremiah	Hebrew	Exalted of the Lord	
Jeremy	Hebrew	God will uplift, appointed by God	
Jesse	Hebrew	Wealthy	

Jesus	Hebrew	God will help	
Joakim	Hebrew	The Lord will judge	Joachim, Jochen, Johann
Joel	Hebrew	God is willing, Jehovah is the Lord	
John	Hebrew	God is merciful	John, Jonny, Johnny, Jonathan, Juan, Shane, Sean, Jack, Ian, Iain, Ivan, Iwan
Jonah	Hebrew	A dove	
Jonathan	Hebrew	God gives	
Jordan	Hebrew	To descend, to flow	
Jorgen	Hebrew	Farmer	Jürgen
Joseph	Hebrew	God will increase	Jose, Joey, Josef, Ioseph, Iosef, Giuseppe, Joe, Sepp, Joseph, Joze, Yusuf
Joshua	Hebrew	Jehovah saves	Josh
Josiah	Hebrew	Fire of the Lord	
Judd	Hebrew	Praised	
Jude	Hebrew	Praise	
Justin	Hebrew	Just, true	
Kabos	Hebrew	Swindler	
Kaniel	Hebrew	Stalk, reed	
Kenan	Hebrew	Possession	
Label	Hebrew	Lion	
Lazarus	Hebrew	God's help	Lazre, Lazar, Lazaro, Laszlo, El'azar, Lázár
Lemuel	Hebrew	Devoted to God, beloging to God	
Leshem	Hebrew	Precious stone	
Levi	Hebrew	United	Lev
Malachi	Hebrew	Messenger of God	Malachy, Malachai
Mario	Hebrew	Bitter, king-ruler	Marius, Marion

Matai	Hebrew	Gift of God	Matteo, Matthäus, Mateus, Mateo, Matthew, Matthias, Matias, Matia, Mattias, Matze, Mathew, Mathias, Matthias, Mattieu, Matheu, Matyus, Matthuas, Mathern, Mayhew, Mattheson, Matthieson, Matthews, Mattheus, Mathe, Mattison, Massey, Matt, Matty, Mats, Máté, Mátyás
Mayer	German, Latin, Hebrew	Farmer; greater; bringer of light	Meyer, Meir, Meier, Mayr, Myer, Mayor, Myerson
Mehetabel	Hebrew	Favoured by God, God is doing good	Mehitabel, Mehitabelle, Metabel, Hetty, Hitty
Mendel	Hebrew, Middle English	Wisdom; repairer	Mel, Mendelssohn, Menachem, Menahem

Michael	Hebrew	Who is like God	Michail, Mikhail, Mikas, Mikel, Michel, Miguel, Michelangelo, Micah, Michiel, Micha, Mischa, Mitchell, Mitch, Michau, Mikkel, Michel, Michele, Mihon, Mikhos, Mihal, Mick, Mickey, Micky, Mike, Mikey, Mickie, Midge, Mihály, Mikó
Mihaly	Hebrew	Who is like God?	
Mordecai	Hebrew	Warrior	Mordechai, Mort, Mordy, Morty
Moses	Hebrew, Egyptian, Greek	Saved; child; taken from water	Mose, Moe, Mosya, Moey, Moss, Moshe, Moishe, Mosheh, Moyes, Moyse
Nachmanke	Hebrew	Compassionate one, one who comforts	
Nadav	Hebrew	Nobel, a generous one	
Nathaniel	Hebrew	Gift of God	Nathanael, Nathan, Nataniel, Natan, Nate, Nat, Natty
Nehemiah	Hebrew	God's compassion	Nemiah
Nirel	Hebrew	God's field	Niriel, Niria, Nira, Nir, Nyree
Noadiah	Hebrew	God assembles	

Noah	Hebrew	Comfort, wanderer	Noa, Noe, Noach, Noel, Noam
Obadiah	Hebrew	Servant of God	Obed, Obie, Obe
Omar	Arabic, Hebrew, German	First son, disciple; gifted speaker; famous	Omer
Oran	Gaelic, Hebrew	Pale one; pine	Orin, Orren, Oren, Orran, Orrin, Oram, Orrie
Oren	Hebrew, Gaelic	Ash-tree, pale; pine tree	
Osaze	Hebrew	Favoured by God	
Osborne	Hebrew	Soldier of God	
Oz	Hebrew	Strength	Ozzy, Ozzie
Palti	Hebrew	My escape	
Ranen	Hebrew	Joyous	
Raphael	Hebrew	Healed by God	Rafael, Rafaelle, Rafaello, Rafe, Rafer, Rafi, Raff, Raph, Rafferty, Rafal
Ravid	Hebrew	Wander	
Reuben	Hebrew	Behold, a son	Rube, Ruben, Reubin, Rubin, Reuven, Reuby, Ben, Benny
Reuel	Hebrew	Friend of God	
Rishon	Hebrew	First	
Roni	Hebrew	Shout for joy, my song of joy	
Ruben	Hebrew	Behold, a son	
Sachiel	Hebrew	Angel of water	
Sagiv	Hebrew	Mighty, with strength	

Saloman	Hebrew	Peaceful	Salomi, Solomon, Schlomo, Shlomo, Soloman, Salomon, Salmon, Sholem, Shalom, Solom, Salamon
Sam	Hebrew	To hear	
Samson	Hebrew	Like the sun, his ministry	Sampson, Sanson, Sansone, Sam, Sammy
Samuel	Hebrew	His name is God	Samuele, Samuelson, Samelle, Sam, Sammy, Sammie, Shemuel, Schmuel, Shem
Saul	Hebrew	Asked for	Sol, Sauly, Solly
Seff	Hebrew	A wolf	
Seraphim	Hebrew	Burning ones, angels, ardent	
Seth	Hebrew	Appointed one	Sethia
Shulamith	Hebrew	Peaceful	Shulamit
Simon	Hebrew	He who hears	Simeon, Siomonn, Sim, Shimon, Semjén
Sivan	Hebrew	The ninth month	
Talman	Hebrew	Io injure, to oppress	
Teman	Hebrew	Right hand, south	
Temani	Hebrew	Of Teman	
Timur	Hebrew, Hungarian, Turkish	Iron	Tomor, Tömör
Tivon	Hebrew	Lover of nature	

Tobias	Hebrew	God is good	Tobia, Tobiah, Toby, Tobit, Tobin, Tova, Tobey, Tóbiás
Tovi	Hebrew	Good	
Udeh	Hebrew	Praise	
Uri	Hebrew	Light	Urie
Uriel	Hebrew	Light of God	Uriell
Yadon	Hebrew	He will judge	
Yakov	Hebrew, Russian	The supplanter, held by the heel	
Yan	Hebrew	God's grace	Yann, Yannic, Yanni
Yanis	Hebrew	God's gift	Yannis
Yarin	Hebrew	To understand	
Yehudi	Hebrew	Praise God, a man from Judah, a Jew	Yehuda
Zabulon	Hebrew	To exhalt, honor	
Zaccheo	Hebrew	The one God remembers	Zaccheus
Zachary	Hebrew	God remembers, renowned by God	Zacharias, Zakary, Zacarius, Zaccaria, Zachariah, Zechairah, Zackry, Zach, Zack, Zak, Zacharie, Zaccaria, Zacharyah
Zakai	Aramaic, Hebrew	Innocent, one who is pure	Zakkai
Zane	Hebrew, Old English	God's grace, sea-friend	Zain
Zazu	Hebrew	Movement	
Zebulon	Hebrew	Home	
Zedekiah	Hebrew	Justice of the lord	Zed
Zephan	Hebrew	Treasured by God	

Zev	Hebrew, Hindu	Deer, wolf	Zvi, Zevie, Zivia, Ziva, Zeva
Ziff	Hebrew	Wolf	
Zion	Hebrew	A sign	
Ziv	Hebrew	Very bright	

Hindu Male Baby Names

Name	Origin	Meaning	Similiar Names
Aakarshan	Hindu	Attraction	
Abhay	Hindu	A son of Dharma	
Abhijit	Hindu	A constellation dear to Hari	
Achyuta	Hindu	A name of Vishnu	
Aditya	Hindu	Lord of the sun	
Ajatashatru	Hindu	A name of Vishnu	
Akaash	Hindu	Sky	
Akshay	Hindu	Name of a God	
Amar	Hindu	Forever	
Amit	Hindu	Endless	
Amrit	Hindu	Nectar	
Amulya	Hindu	Priceless	
Anand	Hindu	Bliss, happiness	Ananda
Angada	Hindu	A son of Lakshmana	
Anjuman	Hindu	A party place (mehfil)	
Anniruddha	Hindu	Son of Pradyummna	
Anoop	Hindu	Incomparable, the best	
Arjun	Hindu	One of the Pandavas	
Ashish	Hindu	Blessings	
Ashwin	Hindu	Strong horse	
Asija	Hindu	A great sage, brother of Brihaspati	
Asuman	Hindu	Lord of vital breaths	
Asvathama	Hindu	Sun of Drona	
Asvin	Hindu	(Nasatya and Dasra) Gods of medicine	
Atharvan	Hindu	Knower of the Arthara vedas	
Atilla	Hungarian	Beloved father	
Atmajyoti	Hindu	Light of Atma	

Atman	Hindu	The self	
Balavan	Hindu	Powerful	
Bali	Hindu	Mighty warrior	Balin, Balik
Bhrigu	Hindu	A Prajapati	
Bhudev	Hindu	Lord of the Earth	
Bod	Hungarian	Branch	Bodony
Chander	Hindu	Moon	
Dahana	Hindu	A Rudra	
Darshan	Hindu	A God's name	
Dattatreya	Hindu	A son of Atri, a God	
Devarsi	Hindu	Sage of the Devas	
Dhananjay	Hindu	Arjuna	
Dharuna	Hindu	A rishi	
Dhatri	Hindu	A son of Vishnu, Lakshmi	
Dilip	Hindu	A king, ancestor of Rama	Deleep
Duranjaya	Hindu	A heroic son	
Durga	Hindu	Unreachable	
Durjaya	Hindu	Difficult to conquer	
Ekachakra	Hindu	Son of Kashyapa	
Eknath	Hindu	Poet, saint	
Falgun	Hindu	Month in the Hindu calendar	Phalgun
Ganesh	Hindu	A Hindu God	
Gopal	Hindu	Lord Krishna	
Harsh	Hindu	Joy	
Hastin	Hindu	Elephant	

Hungarian Male Baby Names

Name	Origin	Meaning	Similiar Names
Aba	Hungarian	Father	Abod, Abony
Asztrik	Hungarian	Made from ashenwood	
Atilla	Hungarian	Beloved father	
Bajnok	Hungarian	Victor	
Bars	Hungarian	Pepper	Bors
Becse	Hungarian	The kite	
Bence	Hungarian	Victor	
Beriszl	Hungarian	Honor	
Bod	Hungarian	Branch	Bodony
Bodor	Hungarian	Curly	
Botond	Hungarian	Mace wielding warrior	
Csaba	Hungarian	From mythology, sheperd, wanderer	
Cseke	Hungarian	Puller, carrier	
Csepel	Hungarian	Young forest	
Csongor	Hungarian	Hunting bird	
Deli	Hungarian	Warrior	
Denes	Greek, Hungarian	Wine, drama	
Domokos	Hungarian	God's own	Domonkos, Domos
Egyed	Hungarian	Shieldbearer	
Elek	Hungarian	Helper and defender of mankind	
Farkas	Hungarian	Wolf	
Ferenc	Latin, Hungarian	Independent, free	
Fodor	Hungarian	Curly haired	
Folkus	Hungarian	People, famous	
Frigyes	Hungarian	Peace, might	
Gara	Hungarian	Goshawk	
Gedeon	Hungarian	Warrior, devastator	
Gerzson	Hungarian	Stranger, banished	Gerson
Gyula	Hungarian	Name of a honor	
Halian	Zuni Indian	Of Julius	
Hont	Hungarian	Dogbreeder, friend of dogs	
Hunor	Hungarian	A name of an etnhic group	

Kalman	Hungarian	Strong and manly	
Kaplony	Hungarian	Tiger	
Kardos	Hungarian	Swordsman	
Karsa	Hungarian	Falcon	
Kartal	Hungarian	Eagle	
Keleman	Hungarian	Gentle, kind	Kelemen
Kemenes	Hungarian	Furnace maker	
Kende	Hungarian	Hame of a honor	
Kerecsen	Hungarian	Falcon	
Kers	Todas Indian	Name of a plant	
Keve	Hungarian	Pebble	
Kolos	Hungarian	Scholar	
Kund	Hungarian	A name of a honor	
Laborc	Hungarian	Brave panther	
Ladomér	Hungarian	Trapper	
Lantos	Hungarian	Lute player	
László	Hungarian	Might, fame	
Lehel	Hungarian	Breathes	
Lél	Hungarian	Bugler	
Len	Hopi Indian, Scandinavian	Flute, with a lion's hart	Lenny
Levente	Hungarian	Being	
Lipót	Hungarian	Brave	
Loránd	Hungarian	Brave warrior	Lóránt
Lõrinc	Hungarian	Laurentian	
Marót	Hungarian	Moravian	
Medárd	Hungarian	Great, strong	
Megyer	Hungarian	Hungarian	Magyar
Menyhért	Hungarian	Royal light	
Miksa	Hungarian	Similar to God	
Milán	Hungarian	Kind	
Mór	Hungarian	Moorish	Móric, Moore
Nyék	Hungarian	Borderlands	
Odon	Hungarian	Wealthy protector	
Odön	Hungarian	Keeper of the fief	Ödön
Oguz	Hungarian	Arrow	
Ompoly	Hungarian	Ampleumian	
Ond	Hungarian	Tenth child	
Orbán	Hungarian	Citydweller, educated man	Orbó, Oros
Orkény	Hungarian	Frightening man	Örkény
Ormos	Hungarian	Like a cliff	
Ors	Hungarian	Man, hero	Örs
Ozor	Hungarian	Name of an ethnic group	

Ozséb	Hungarian	Pious	Özséb
Ozsvát	Hungarian	Deity, might	
Pázmán	Hungarian	Right, man	
Pellegrin	Hungarian	Pilgrim	
Pentele	Hungarian	Merciful, lion	
Pongor	Hungarian	All might	Pongrác
Radomér	Hungarian	Happy, peace	
Rendor	Hungarian	Policeman	
Robi	Hungarian	Shining with fame	
Sandor	Hungarian	Helper and defender of mankind	
Sebes	Hungarian	Fast	
Solt	Hungarian	Name of an honor	
Sólyom	Hungarian	Falcon	
Soma	Hungarian	A kind of berry	
Surány	Hungarian	Name of an honor	
Szemere	Hungarian	Small man, demolisher	
Szervác	Hungarian	Freed	
Szevér	Hungarian	Serious, strict	Szörény
Taksony	Hungarian	Well fed, content,merciliess,wild	
Tardos	Hungarian	Bald	
Tarján	Hungarian	Name of an honor	
Tas	Hungarian	Well fed,stone	
Tétény	Hungarian	Chieftain	Töhötöm
Tihamér	Hungarian	Likes silence	
Timur	Hebrew, Hungarian, Turkish	Iron	Tomor, Tömör
Titusz	Hungarian	Dove, honored	
Tivadar	Hungarian	Gift of God	
Tomaj	Hungarian	Name of a clan	
Ugod	Hungarian	Name of a clan	
Ugor	Hungarian	Hungarian	Ugron
Uros	Hungarian	Little lord	
Uzor	Hungarian	Name of an ethnic group	Ozor
Várkony	Hungarian	Name of an Avar ethnic group	
Varsàny	Hungarian	Name of an ethnic group	
Vayk	Hungarian	Rich	
Vidor	Hungarian	Happy	
Vitéz	Hungarian	Brave warrior	
Yakecan	Dene Indian	Sky, song	
Zádor	Hungarian	Violent	
Zalán	Hungarian	Thrower, hitter	

Zámor	Hungarian	Plough-land	
Zaránd	Hungarian	Gold	
Zerind	Hungarian	Serb	
Zobor	Hungarian	Gathering	
Zoltán	Hungarian	Chieftain	
Zombor	Hungarian	Buffalo	Zsombor
Zorán	Hungarian	Dawn	
Zsolt	Hungarian	Name of an honor	

Irish Male Baby Names

Name	Origin	Meaning	Similiar Names
Galvin	Irish	Sparrow	
Gannon	Irish	Fair-complexioned	
Laoghaire	Irish	Calf herder, a shepard	
Liam	Irish	Unwavering protector	
Mac	Scottish, Irish, English	Son of	
Moriarty	Irish	Sea warrior	
Nevan	Irish	Holy, little saint	
Quinlan	Irish	Well-shaped, athletic	
Shane	Irish	God is gracious	
Shea	Irish	Hawk-like, stately	Shay
Sheridon	Irish	Wild one	Sheridan
Sinead	female	Irish	gracious

Italian Male Baby Names

Name	Origin	Meaning	Similiar Names
Dante	Italian	Lasting	
Napoleon	Greek, Italian	Lion of the woods; from the city of Naples	Nappie, Nappy, Nap, Leon, Leo
Nino	Italian	God is gracious	Ninoshka
Pancrazio	Italian	Supreme ruler, all powerful	
Primo	Italian	First one	Prime
Rocco	Italian	Rest	
Romeo	Italian	Pilgrim to Rome	Rome, Roman, Romain
Santo	Italian	A saint	Santos
Taddeo	Italian	Courageous, one who praises	
Tancredo	Italian	Of thoughtful counsel	Tancrede
Ugo	Italian	Bright in mind and spirit	
Zanebono	Italian	The good one	
Zanipolo	Italian	Little gift of God	

Japanese Male Baby Names

Name	Origin	Meaning	Similiar Names
Botan	Japanese	Peony	
Haru	Japanese	Born in the spring	
Hiroshi	Japanese	Generous	
Jiro	Japanese	Second male	
Kanaye	Japanese	Zealous one	
Kin	Japanese	Golden	
Kisho	Japanese	One who knows his own mind	
Kiyoshi	Japanese	Quiet	
Mamoru	Japanese	Earth	Mamo
Masakazu	Japanese	First son of Masa	
Raidon	Japanese	Thunder God	
Ringo	Japanese	Apple, peace be with you	
Ronin	Japanese	Samurai without a master	
Ryoichi	Japanese	First son of Ryo	
Ryozo	Japanese	Third son of Ryo	
Ryuichi	Japanese	First son of Ryu	
Ryuji	Japanese	Dragon Man	
Seiichi	Japanese	First son of Sei	
Senichi	Japanese	First son of Sen	
Shigekazu	Japanese	First son of Shige	
Shinichi	Japanese	First son of Shin	
Shoichi	Japanese	First son of Sho	
Shuichi	Japanese	First son of Shu	
Shunichi	Japanese	First son of Shun	
Taro	Japanese	First-born male	
Tomo	Japanese	A twin	
Yasuo	Japanese	Peaceful one	
Yogi	Japanese	One of the yoga practice	
Yoshi	Japanese	Better, best	
Yukio	Japanese	Gets what he wants, God will nourish	

Korean Male Baby Names

Name	*Origin*	*Meaning*	*Similiar Names*
Bae	Korean	Inspiration	
Chin	Korean	Precious	
Jin	Chinese, Korean	Gold; truth, treasure, pearl	
Joo-Chan	Korean	Praise the Lord	
Jung	Korean	Righteous	
Seung	Korean	Successor, winning	

Latin Male Baby Names

Name	Origin	Meaning	Similiar Names
Abundiantus	Latin	Plentiful	Abbondanzio, Abbondazio, Abbondio
Acario	Latin	Ungrateful	Acharius
Accursius	Latin	To hasten	Accorso, Accursio
Ace	Latin	Unity, one, first rate	
Acuzio	Latin	Sharp	
Adalrico	Latin, Old German	Noble, powerful and rich	Adalricus, Adalrich
Adelais	Latin	Noble	Adelasia
Adeodatus	Latin	Given by God	Adeodato, Adiodato
Adiran	Latin	Of the Adriatic	
Adrian	Greek, Latin	Rich, wealthy, dark one	Adrien, Adrie, Hadrian, Adrianus, Adriano, Hadrianus
Afro	Latin	From Africa	Africano
Alban	Latin	White, fair	Alben, Albin, Albion, Albano
Albion	Latin	Blond	Albione
Amadeus	Latin	Love of god	Amado, Amadis
Amado	Latin	Loving deity	
Antal	Latin	Prince	

Anthony	Latin, Greek	Priceless, flourishing, flower	Anthoney, Antonius, Anton, Antony, Antonio, Tony, Toni, Tonio, Tonie, Tone, Tee, Toney, Antonio, Anthony, Antone, Antoine, Anth, Nee
Arley	Latin	The bowman	
Auburn	Latin	Fair	Alban, Aubin
Augustus	Latin	Exalted	Augustin, Augustine, Augustina, Augie, August, Augusta, Gus, Gussy, Gussie, Gusta, Austin, Agustin, Agostino, Augusto
Aurelio	Latin	Gold	Aurelius, Aurilius, Aurilio
Balbo	Latin	Inarticulate	
Balint	Latin	Strong and healthy	
Baran	Latin	Form of star Aldebaran	
Barber	Latin	Beard	Barbour
Benedict	Latin	Blessed	Benedetto, Bennett, Benet, Benner, Benoit, Benn, Bent, Benton, Bengt, Benen, Bene, Benedekt
Benito	Latin	Blessed	Ben
Blaise	Latin	Stammerer	Biagio, Blase, Blaze, Blis
Boone	Latin, French	Good	Bono

Branch	Latin	Extension	
Braz	Latin	Stammerer	
Brencis	Latin	Crowned with laurel	
Brutus	Latin	Bruto	
Calixto	Latin	A chalice	
Callis	Latin	Cup	Callys
Carey	Latin	Dear, pleasant stream	Cary, Carry, Carrie, Kerry, Kerrie
Cassius	Latin	Vain	
Cato	Latin	Sagacious, wise one	
Ceasar	Latin	To cut	
Ceasar	Latin	Hairy child, long haired	Cesar, Cezar
Chauncey	Latin	Chancellor	
Chester	Latin	Camp	Chet, Ches, Chess
Ciceron	Latin	Chickpea	Cicero, Ciro, Cecero
Clarence	Latin	Clear, bright	Claron, Clarendon
Clement	Latin	Merciful	Clements, Clemens, Clemmons, Clemon, Clem, Klemens
Comfort	Latin	Strengthen	
Constantine	Latin	Faithful, firmness	Konstantin
Cooper	Latin	Cask, barrel maker	Coop
Cordell	Latin	Small rope	Cord, Cordas, Cordie, Cordy
Cornelius	Latin	Horn	Cornell, Cornel
Crispin	Latin	Curly	Crispen, Crispus, Crispo, Krispen, Crisp
Curtis	Latin, Old French	Court, courteous	Curt, Curtys
Dean	Latin, Old English	Presiding official, valley	

Delmore	Latin	Sea	Del, Delmar, Delmer
Desiderio	Latin, French	So long hoped for, crave, desire	Desi
Desmond	Celtic, Latin	Man of the world, society	Desi, Des
Dexter	Latin	Dexterous, right side	
Dominic	Latin	Of the Lord	Dominick, Domenico, Dominica, Dominique, Dominik, Domingo, Dominy, Dom, Nick
Donatien	French, Latin	Gift	Donato
Drake	Old English, Latin	Ale duck, dragon	
Duke	Latin	Leader	
Durand	Latin	Enduring	Durandt, Durante, Durant, Duran
Ellery	German/Latin	One who lives near the elder tree, cheerful	Elery, Ellory, Elory, Ellary, Elary
Estes	Latin	Estuary	Eston
Ethan	Hebrew/Latin	Strong, firm, constant	Ethen, Etan
Fabian	Latin	Bean	Fabius, Fab, Fabyan, Fabio
Farrar	Latin	Blacksmith	Farar, Farron, Faron, Farrier
Februus	Latin	Pagan God	Feb, Febby
Felix	Latin	Happy	Felice
Ferenc	Latin, Hungarian	Independent, free	
Ferris	Celtic, Latin	Rock, iron	Ferrys, Ferrell, Ferrel
Fitz	Latin	Son	Fitzgerald, Fitzroy, Fitzhugh, Fitzpatrick

Francis	Latin, Old French	From France, free	Frank, Frankie, Franz, Franco, Ferenc, Franci
Galloway	Latin	From Gaul	Galway
Garner	Latin	Granary	
Garnet	Latin	Red seed	Garnett
Gary	Old English, Latin, Teutonic	Spear carrier	Garry, Garrie, Garvey, Garvie, Garvin, Gervis, Gervais, Gervase, Garrick
Gram	Latin	Grain	
Grant	Latin	Great	
Gregory	Latin	Vigilant watch	Gergely, Grzegorz
Hector	Latin	Anchor, steadfast	
Ignacio	Latin	One who is lively	Ignatios, Ignazio, Ignazios, Ignatius
Ilias	Latin	Jehovah is my God	
Ince	Latin	Innocent	
Javan	Latin	Angel of Greece	
Jerolin	Latin	Holy name	
Julian	Latin	Youthful	Jules, Julius, Jul, Julio
Justus	Latin	Justice	Justice, Just, Jussey
Kasen	Latin	Protected with a helmet	
Kester	Latin	From the camp of the Roman army	
Korvin	Latin	Crow	Corvin
Lamberto	Latin	Wealthy in land, brilliant	Lambert

Lawrence	Latin	Laurel crown	Laurence, Lawrance, Lorenz, Loren, Laurens, Lorin, Lorcan, Lon, Lonnie, Loring, Lawford, Lawley, Lawton, Lawler, Laughton, Lawry, Larry, Laurent, Lorenzo, Lauritz, Lorne, Lawson, Lars, Larson, Larkin, Labhras
Lester	Latin	Legion camp	Les
Luke	Latin	Bringer of light	Luc, Lucas, Luckas, Luchas, Luca, Luka, Lukas, Lucais, Lucan, Lucian, Lucien, Lucius, Luciano, Lukyan, Lukian, Lukács
Mace	Latin	Aromatic spice	
Magnus	Latin, Scandinavian	Large; the great	Manus, Magnuson, Magnum
Major	Latin	Greater	Majeur, Majors, Majorie

Mark	Latin	Warlike, hammer, defender	Marek, Marc, Marcus, Markus, Marcel, Marceau, Marque, Marco, Marek, Marko, Marus, Markos, Marks, Marx, March, Marius, Marquette, Marquis, Marky, Markie, Marilo, Márk, Markó, Márkus
Martin	Latin	Of Mars	Marten, Martyn, Marton, Martino, Martins, Marty, Martie, Mart, Mertin, Mertil, Martinson, Martel, Martinet, Martinique, Márton
Maurice	French, Latin, Old English	Moorish; dark; moor land	Morris, Morse, Maury, Morry, Morey, Morrie, Moritz, Moriz, Morets, Meuriz, Moss, Morrell, Mauricio, Maurizio, Murray, Maryse, Morrison

Max	Latin	The greatest	Maximilien, Maximiliano, Maximus, Maxim, Maximo, Maxfield, Maximino, Maximilian, Maxey, Maxie, Mac, Maxa, Mack, Maks, Maksim, Massimiliano
Mayer	German, Latin, Hebrew	Farmer; greater; bringer of light	Meyer, Meir, Meier, Mayr, Myer, Mayor, Myerson
Miles	Latin, Old German, Greek	Soldier; merciful; millstone	Myles, Milo, Milos, Milan, Milah, Miles, Mila
Miner	Latin	Youth	
Monte	Latin	Moutain	Monty
Morris	Latin	Dark skinned	Maurice, Morrie, Morry, Morse, Moss, Morrison
Narciso	Latin	A lily, daffodil	
Nemo	Latin	No name, nobody	
Nigel	Latin	Dark one	
Nimbus	Latin	Rain cloud, halo	
Noble	Latin	Honorable one, well born	Nobel, Nobile
Nona	Latin	Ninth	
Octavius	Latin	Eighth child	Octavus, Octavio, Octavian, Tavie, Tavy, Oktávián
Oliver	Old Norse, Latin, Old French	Kind one; olive tree, peace	Olivier, Olivero, Olley, Olly, Ollie, Noll, Nolly

Orion	Latin, Greek	Dawn, east; son of fire, the hunter	Orien, Oris
Orlando	Latin	Bright sun	Orly, Lando
Orson	Old English, Latin	Spearman's son; bear	Orsen, Orsin, Orsini, Sonny
Ossian	Latin	Fawn	
Ovid	Latin	Lamb	
Patrick	Latin	Noble one	Patrice, Padraic, Padraig, Padruig, Pat, Paddy, Patterson, Paterson, Pattison, Rick, Ricky
Paul	Latin	Little one	Pol, Pawl, Pablo, Paolo, Pauly, Pauley, Pawley, Pavel, Paulin, Pavlo, Paulo, Paulus, Powell, Pál
Peril	Latin	A trial or test	
Peter	Latin	Rock, stone	Pete, Petey, Pietor, Pytor, Petr, Pieter, Piotr, Pietro, Pedro, Pierre, Piers, Pierce, Peer, Pero, Piero, Peder, Per, Pelle, Peadair, Petrus, Peterson, Perrin, Perkin, Perkins, Parnell, Parle, Parkin, Parkinson, Petrie, Petri, Pierson, Péter, Petõ, Petúr, Pyotr
Placido	Latin	Tranquility	
Pryor	Latin	Head of the priory	Prior

Quentin	Latin	Fifth-born child	Quinton, Quenten, Quenton, Quintin, Quent, Quint, Quinto, Quintilian, Quintus
Rainier	Latin	Ruler	Rainer, Raner
Ransom	Old English, Latin	Son of the shield; redeemer	Ransome, Ranson, Rankin, Rance
Regis	Latin	Kingly, regal	
Remus	Latin	Swift oarsman	
Renee	Latin	Reborn	Rene, Rennie, Renny, Renato, René
Rex	Latin	King	Rei, Roi, Rexford, Rexer
Rivers	Latin, French	Stream of water	River, Rio
Rufus	Latin	Red-haired one	Ruphus, Rufe, Ruff, Rufford
Sebastian	Latin	Revered one	Sebastien, Bastien, Bastian, Sebestyén
Septimus	Latin	Seventh born	
Serge	Latin	Attendant	Sergius, Sergei, Sergio
Silas	Latin	Wood	
Silvester	Latin	Woodman	Sylvester, Sly, Sylvestro, Silvestre, Silvanus, Silas, Syl, Sil, Szilveszter
Silvio	Latin	Belonging to the forest, silver	
Sol	Latin	The sun	Solly
Tanicus	Latin		
Taurin	Latin	Born under the sign of Taurus	

Terence	Latin	Polished, tender	Terrence, Terance, Terencio, Terentius, Terry, Teri, Terris
Thaddeaus	Latin	Couragues, praiser	Thaddeus, Thaddaus, Thaddea, Thada, Taddeo, Tadeo, Tadeusz, Tadgh, Thad, Taddy, Tadda, Tad, Ted, Thadea
Trent	Latin, Old English	Torrent, dweller by the Trent	Trenton
Trenus	Latin		
Tristan	Old Welsh, Latin	Noisy one, laborer	Tristram
Tyrus	Latin	Person from Tyre	Ty
Ulysses	Latin	The hateful one, wounded in the thigh	Ulises, Uilioc
Urban	Latin	From the city	Urbano, Urbanus, Urbaine, Urbane
Valentin	Latin	Good health	Valentino, Valente
Valeray	Old French, Latin	Valor, strong	
Vernon	French, Latin	Alder tree, springlike	Vern, Verda, Verne, Verney, Verna, Vernia, Vernis, Virna, Vernal, Laverne, Lavinia
Victor	Latin	Victor	Viktor, Vitorio, Vittorio, Vick, Vic, Vince
Vincent	Latin	Conquering	Vinko

Virgil	Latin	Unknown	
Vito	Latin	Conquerer	
Zaniel	Latin	Angel of Mondays	
Zanobi	Latin	Scarcely alive	

Native American Male Names

Name	Origin	Meaning	Similiar Names
Adriel	Native American	Beaver, symbol of skill	
Akando	Native American	Ambush	
Ali	Arabic, Native American	God, little, the highest	Allah
Anoki	Native American	An actor	
Delsin	Native American	He is so	
Dyami	Native American	Eagle	
Elu	Native American	Full of grace	
Helaku	Native American	Sunny day	
Jacy	Native American	The moon	
Jolon	Native American	Valley of the dead oaks	
Len	Hopi Indian, Scandinavian	Flute, with a lion's heart	Lenny
Motega	Native American	New arrow	
Nalren Nantan Nodin	Dene Indian Apache Indian Native American	Thawed out Spokesman Wind	
Paco	Native American, Spanish	Bald eagle; a free man	
Patamon	Native American	Raging	
Pilan	Native American	Supreme essence	
Sahale	Native American	Above	
Shaman	Native American	Holy man	Schamane
Tyee	Native American	Chief	
Wyome	Native American	Plain	
Yahto	Native American	Blue	
Yancy	Native American	Yankee	Yank
Yuma	Native American	Son of the chief	

Nigerian Male Baby Names

Name	*Origin*	*Meaning*	*Similiar Names*
Ajayi	Yoruban, Nigerian	Born face-down	
Aren	Nigerian	Eagle	
Bem	Nigerian	Peace	
Daren	Nigerian	Born at night	
Odion	Nigerian	First of twins	

Norse Male Baby Names

Name	Origin	Meaning	Similiar Names
Floke	Teutonic, Norse	Guardian of the people	
Gamble	Norse	Old	
Gareth	Welsh, Norse, Old French	Gentle; enclosure; watchful	Garth, Garret, Garrett, Garreth, Gareth, Garit, Gary, Garry, Gar
Geir	Norse	Spear	
Hakan	Norse, Turkish	Noble, fiery	
Igor	Norse	Hero	
Kelby	Old Norse	From the farm by the springs	
Kerr	Norse	Marshland	Keir, Kirby
Kirk	Old Norse	From the church	Kirkley, Kirkwood, Kirby, Kurk, Kirkus
Lamont	Norse	Lawyer	
Lang	Old English, Old Norse	Long, tall	Langdon, Langford, Langley, Langston, Langhorne, Langtry
Leif	Old Norse	Beloved	
Magne	Norse	Fierce warrior	
Oddvar	Norse	The spear's point	
Odin	Norse	Head God in Norse mythology	
Olaf	Old Norse	Talisman, ancestor	Olav, Olof, Olin, Olen, Olie

Oliver	Old Norse, Latin, Old French	Kind one; olive tree, peace	Olivier, Olivero, Olley, Olly, Ollie, Noll, Nolly
Oscar	Old Norse	Divine spear	Osgood, Oskar, Oszkár
Ragnar	Norse	A wise leader	
Raynard	Old German, Old Norse	Brave one; mighty army	Raynard, Renard, Reinhard, Raynor, Reinhart, Rinehart, Renaud, Reynaud, Reynart, Reyner, Rey
Ronald	Old Norse	Mighty	Ronnie, Ronny, Ron, Renaldo, Ronan, Naldo
Roscoe	Old Norse	From the deer forest	
Skipp	Old Norse	Ship owner	skipper, skippy, skip
Sutherland	Norse	From the southern land	Sutton, Sutcliff, Suffield, Sundy
Terje	Norse	Of Thor's spear	
Thor	Old Norse	Thunder	Thorbert, Thordis, Tor, Soren, Sören, Søren
Thurston	Norse	Thor's stone	Thurstin, Turstan
Torsten	Norse	The stone of Thor	
Turpin	Old Norse	Thunder-Finn	
Yngvar	Norse	Of Ing's army	Ingvarr

Norwegian Male Baby Names

Name	Origin	Meaning	Similiar Names
Aricin	Norwegian	The eternal kings son	
Arkin	Norwegian	The eternal king's son	
Canute	Norwegian	Knot	
Carr	Norwegian	From the marsh	
Dag	Norwegian	Day	Dagney, Dagny, Dagget, Day, Dayton, Daymond
Egil	Norwegian, French	The edge or point, a sting	
Einar	Norwegian	Warrior, leader	
Finn	Norwegian	Laplander	
Ivar	Norwegian	Archer, a norse God	

Persian Male Baby Names

Name	Origin	Meaning	Similiar Names
Casper	Persian	Treasurer	Caspar
Cyrus	Persian	The sun	Cy
Darius	Persian	King	Dario, Darien, Darian
Jasper	Persian	Treasurer	
Kaspar	Persian	A treasured secret	
Khorshed	Persian	Sun	
Khortdad	Persian	Perfection	
Rashne	Persian	Judge	
Sarosh	Persian	Prayer	
Siamak	Persian	Bringer of joy, great emperor	Sia
Xerxes	Persian	Prince	

Polish Male Baby Names

Name	Origin	Meaning	Similiar Names
Aurek	Polish	Golden-haired	
Bazyli	Polish	Royalty	
Bialy	Polish	White-haired boy	
Dobry	Polish	Good	
Erek	Polish	Lovable	
Gerik	Polish	Prosperous spearman	
Jarek	Polish	Born in January	
Jedrek	Polish	Strong, manly	
Jerzy	Polish	Farmer	
Mandek	Polish	Army man	
Marcin	Polish	Warlike	
Nelek	Polish	Like a horn	
Stanislaw	Polish, Old English	Camp glory; stone clearing	Stanislao, Stanislau, Stanislav, Stanislaus, Stanislav, Sztaniszláv, Stanislas, Stanislavsky, Stan, Aineislis, Stasio
Tanek	Polish	Immortal	

Polynesian Male Baby Names

Name	Origin	Meaning	Similiar Names
Ulani	male	Cheerful	

Russian Male Baby Names

Name	Origin	Meaning	Similiar Names
Boris	Russian	Fight, battler	Bors, Borys
Gavrie	Russian	Man of God	
Sacha	Russian	Helper and defender of mankind	Sasha, Sascha
Yakov	Hebrew, Russian	The supplanter, held by the heel	
Yerik	Russian	Appointed by God	

Sanskrit Male Baby Names

Name	Origin	Meaning	Similiar Names
Rajiv	Sanskrit	Striped	
Ramesh	Sanskrit	Ruler of Rama	
Veda	Sanskrit	Eternal knowledge	Vedis

Saxon Male Baby Names

Name	Origin	Meaning	Similiar Names
Aiken	Anglo-Saxon	Sturdy, oaken	
Alston	Anglo-Saxon	From the old manor	Alton
Anson	Anglo-Saxon	Son of a nobleman, son of Ann or Hans	Ansen, Ansonia, Hansen, Hanson
Archibald	Anglo-Saxon	Bold prince	Arch, Archie, Archy, Arkady, Arky
Bardon	Anglo-Saxon	Barley valley	
Berkeley	Anglo-Saxon	From the birch meadow	Berkley
Braxton	Anglo-Saxon	Brock's town	
Byron	French, Anglo-Saxon	From the cottage, bear	Byram, Byran
Daley	Gaelic, Anglo-Saxon	Assembly, from the valley	Dailey, Daily
Eamon	Anglo-saxon	Wealthy guardian	Amon
Garett	Anglo-Saxon	Powerful with the spear	
Graham	Anglo-Saxon	Warlike	
Irvin	Anglo-Saxon	Lover of the sea	Irv, Irvine
Marvin	Celtic, Anglo-Saxon	Beautiful sea; good friend	Mervin, Mervyn, Merwin, Merwyn, Myrwyn, Murvyn, Myrvyn, Marv
Maynard	Anglo-Saxon	Remarkable strength	
Melville	Anglo-Saxon, Old English	Hillside; town by the mill	Mel

Merlin	Celtic, Anglo-Saxon, Welsh	Sea; falcon; sea hill	Merlyn, Marlin, Marlen, Marwin, Mervin, Merv, Merle
Morton	Anglo-Saxon	City on the moor	Morten, Mortyn, Morty, Mort
Randolph	Anglo-Saxon	Shield, wolf	Randolf, Randall, Randal, Randell, Randl, Randle, Randy, Rankin, Rand, Ran, Randie, Ranulf, Dolf, Dolph
Ross	Scottish, Anglo-Saxon	From the peninsula; horse	Rossano, Roswald
Wystan	Anglo-Saxon	Battle stone	Winston

Scandinavian Male Baby Names

Name	Origin	Meaning	Similiar Names
Gunther	Scandinavian	Battle-army, warrior	Günter, Gunter, Günther
Davin	Scandinavian	Bright finn	
Eric	Scandinavian	Ever-powerful	Erik, Eryk, Erikson
Ingmar	Scandinavian	Famous son	Ingar
Len	Hopi Indian, Scandinavian	Flute, with a lion's hart	Lenny
Lunt	Scandinavian	From the grove	
Quinby	Scandinavian	From the queen's estate	
Magnus	Latin, Scandinavian	Large; the great	Manus, Magnuson, Magnum
Sven	Scandinavian	Youth	Swen, Svend, Svenson, Svensen, Swensen, Swenson

Scottish Male Baby Names

Name	Origin	Meaning	Similiar Names
Alastair	Scottish	Protector of mankind, defender, helper	Alistair, Alistaire, Alastaire, Alister, Alaster, Alasdair
Athol	Scottish	Place name	Avery
Baird	Scottish	Minstrel	Bard
Bairn	Scottish	Child	
Bruce	French, Scottish	Thicket, woodlands	
Camden	Scottish	From the winding valley	
Chalmers	Scottish	Son of the lord	
Dallas	Scottish	Place name, wise	
Davis	Scottish	David's son	
Douglas	Scottish	From the dark water	Douglass, Doug, Dougie, Dugan, Dougal, Dugald
Finlay	Scottish, English	Fair hero, sunbeam	Finn, Finnie, Finny, Finian, Finley, Fyn, Fynn, Finnian
Kenneth	Gaelic, Scottish, Old English	Handsome; born of fire; royal oath	Ken, Kevin, Kennet, Kenny, Kenney, Kenn
Laird	Scottish	Lord, landed gentry	
Leith	Scottish	Wide river	Leathan

Lennox	Scottish	Amid the lems, from the field of elm trees	Lenox, Lenix, Lennie, Lenny, Len
Mac	Scottish, Irish, English	Son of	
Malcom	Scottish	Disciple of Saint Columbia	Mal, Colm
Monroe	Celtic, Scottish	Mouth of the Roe River; wheelwright	Munroe, Munro, Monro
Murdock	Scottish	Victorious at sea	Murdoch, Murtagh
Ogilvy	Old Scottish	From the high peak	Ogilvie, Gil, Gilie, Gilly
Ross	Scottish, Anglo-Saxon	From the peninsula; horse	Rossano, Roswald
Tavis	Scottish	Twin	Tevis, Tav, Tavish, Tamsin

Slavic Male Baby Names

Name	Origin	Meaning	Similiar Names
Bogdan	Slavic	God's gift	
Brodny	Slavic	One who lives near a shallow stream crossing	
Kasimir	Old Slavic	Demands peace	Casmir, Casimir
Miroslav	Slavic	Famous	Miroslaw
Mladen	Slavic	Forever in youth	
Oleg	Slavic	One who is holy	
Radman	Slavic	Joy	
Vencel	Slavic	Wreath, glory	Wenzel, Wazlaw, Vaclav, Venceslas, Vyacheslav
Vladimir	Slavic	To rule with peace, regal	Wolodymyr, Vlad, Vladislav
Wieslav	Slavic	One with great glory	
Ziven	Slavic	Vigorous and alive	
Zorro	Slavic	Golden dawn	

Spanish Male Baby Names

Name	Origin	Meaning	Similiar Names
Abejundio	Spanish	Relating to the abaje (bee)	
Amador	Spanish	Lover	
Amato	Spanish	Beloved	
Amistad	Spanish	Friendship	
Castel	Spanish	Belonging to a castle	
Caton	Spanish	Knowledgable, wise	
Chale	Spanish	Strong and manly	
Ciro	Spanish	The sun	
Colon	Spanish	Dove	
Consuelo	Spanish	Consolation	
Devante	Spanish	Fighter of wrong	Devi, Devan
Diego	Spanish	Saint James	
Emilio	Spanish	Winning one or flatterer	
Esteban	Spanish	Crown	
Fidel	Spanish	Faithful and sincere	Fido, Fidelity
Fonda	Spanish	Profound, well-based	
Galeno	Spanish	Little bright one	
Gaspar	Spanish	Master of treasure	Gaspare, Jasper
Iago	Welsh, Spanish	Supplanter	
Manuel	Spanish	God is with us	Mano, Manolo, Manny, Mani
Neron	Spanish	Strong, stern	
Noe	Spanish	Peace, rest	
Oleos	Spanish	Holy oil used in church	Leo
Paco	Native American, Spanish	Bald eagle; a free man	
Rico	Spanish	Noble ruler	

Rogelio	Spanish	Beautiful one	Ro
Salvador	Spanish	Saviour	Salvatore, Sauveur, Sal
Santiago	Spanish	Supplanter	Santi, Chago, Diego
Senon	Spanish	Given life by Zeus	
Tajo	Spanish	Day	
Ximen	Spanish	Obedient	
Zenon	Spanish	Living	

Swahili Male Baby Names

Name	Origin	Meaning	Similiar Names
Baingana	Swahili	People are equal	
Bakari	Swahili	Promise	
Khairi	Swahili	Kingly	
Rashid	Swahili	Wise adviser	Rasheed

Swedish Male Baby Names

Name	Origin	Meaning	Similiar Names
Axel	Hebrew, Swedish	Divine reward; divine source of life	Axtel
Balder	Swedish	God of light	
Beck	Swedish	Brook	
Bergren	Swedish	Mountain stream	
Bjorn	Swedish	Bear	Björn, Bjorne, Bjarne
Brand	Swedish	Sword blade	
Burr	Swedish	Youth	
Carson	Swedish	Son of Carr	
Denholm	Swedish	Home of the Danes	Denholme, Denby, Denim
Fisk	Swedish	Fisherman	
Greger	Swedish	Vigilant	
Hadrian	Swedish	Dark one	
Staffan	Swedish	A garland	

Teutonic Male Baby Names

Name	Origin	Meaning	Similiar Names
Aimery	Teutonic	Industrious ruler	Aimory
Allard	Old English, Teutonic	Noble and brave	Alard
Archer	Teutonic	The archer	
Bailey	French, English, Teutonic	Bailiff, fortification, able	Baily, Bayley, Bailee, Baylor
Barrett	Teutonic	Bear-like	
Bayard	Old French, Teutonic	Bay horse, red-brown hair	Baylor, Bayless, Baird
Berthold	Teutonic	Glorious ruler	Bertolt, Bertold, Bertholt, Berton
Brant	Teutonic	Firebrand	Brandt
Carl	Teutonic	One who is strong, man	Karl, Karla, Carlton, Carlisle, Carlyle, Carlie, Carly, Carlo, Karlo, Karel, Karoly
Faxon	Teutonic	Long hair	
Floke	Teutonic, Norse	Guardian of the people	
Gary	Old English, Latin, Teutonic	Spear carrier	Garry, Garrie, Garvey, Garvie, Garvin, Gervis, Gervais, Gervase, Garrick

Gerald	Teutonic	Ruler with the spear	Jerold, Jerry, Jerri, Jeri, Jerie, Geri, Gerard, Geraud, Gerardo, Gerhard, Gerhardt, Gerhart, Geraldo, Garold, Gerek, Gerrit, Garrod, Garrard, Gerbert, Girard, Girauld, Girault, Giraut, Gerry, Jerard, Jarett, Jarrett
Gunnar	Teutonic	Bold warrior	
Guy	French, Teutonic	Guide; wood or wide	Gui
Hagan	Teutonic	Strong defence	
Halden	Teutonic	Half Dane	
Hardy	Teutonic	Strong	
Henning	Teutonic	Ruler of an estate	
Holden	Teutonic	Kindly, gracious	
Ingram	Teutonic	King's raven	
Jeffrey	Teutonic	God's peace	Jeff, Jef
Paxton	Teutonic, Old English	Trader; town of peace	
Raeburn	Teutonic	Dweller by the stream where does drink	
Renard	Teutonic	Counselor hard	
Roald	Teutonic	Fame power	
Sigfried	Teutonic	Victory peace	Sigfrid
Sigmund	Teutonic	Victory shield, victory protector	Siegmund, Sigismond, Sigismundo, Siffre, Sigvard, Siggy, Ziggy.

Stewart	Teutonic	Keeper of the estate	Stuart, Steward, Stew, Stu
Theodoric	Teutonic	Ruler of the people	
Thierry	Teutonic	People's ruler	
Thurborn	Teutonic	Dweller by Thor's stream	
Udo	Teutonic	One with great forture, prosperous	
Uland	Teutonic	Noble country	Ulandus
Ulf	Teutonic	Wolf	
Walden	Teutonic	Mighty	
Waldo	Teutonic	Rule	Waldemarr, Waldemar, Waldorf, Walfred, Walden
Warren	Old German, Middle English, Teutonic, French	Watchman, game keeper, enclosure, from La Varenne	Wareine, Warin, Warrener
Wendell	Teutonic	A wend	Wendel, Wedel
Werner	Teutonic	Warin warrior	
Wilbur	Teutonic	Bright resolve	
Willard	Teutonic	Bold resolve	

William	Teutonic	Valiant protector	Wil, Will, Willem, Wilhelm, Wilmos, Wilmot, Wilson, Williams, Williamson, Wills, Willie, Willy, Wiley, Wyley, Wilkie, Willkie, Wilkes, Wylkes, Willis, Wilton, Wilmer, Wilmar, Winton, Willard, Wilford, Guillaume, Guillermo, Vilhelm, Vilem, Viliam, Vasili, Vasily, Uilleam, Uilliam
Wolfgang	Teutonic	Wolf strife	Wolf, Wolfe, Wolfie, Wolcott, Woolsey
Wolfram	Teutonic	Wolf raven	Walram
Yves	Teutonic	Yew, archer	Yvo, Ives, Yvan

Turkish Male Baby Names

Name	Origin	Meaning	Similiar Names
Berk	Turkish	Solid and firm	
Candan	Turkish	Sincerely	
Galip	Turkish	Winner	
Hakan	Norse, Turkish	Noble, fiery	
Selim	Turkish	Peace	
Sevilin	Turkish	Beloved	
Timur	Hebrew, Hungarian, Turkish	Iron	Tomor, Tömör

Ugandan Male Baby Names

Name	Origin	Meaning	Similiar Names
Akello	Ugandan	I have bought	
Bale	Ugandan	Home of the Mutima clan	
Kaikara	Ugandan	Traditional name of God	
Mukasa	Ugandan	God's chief administrator	
Ochen	Ugandan	One of the twins	

Vietnamese Male Baby Names

Name	Origin	Meaning	Similiar Names
Bay	Vietnamese	Born in July, seventh-born son	
Cadeo	Vietnamese	Folk song	
Lam	Vietnamese	Full understanding; knowledge	Lammie, Lammy
Phuoc	Vietnamese	Good luck	
Ritchell	Vietnamese	Nasty, gross	Ritchel, Ratchell
Thai	Vietnamese	Many, multiple	
Tinh	Vietnamese	Mindful; aware	
Tong	Vietnamese	Fragrant	

Welsh Male Baby Names

Name	Origin	Meaning	Similiar Names
Arthus	Welsh	Bear hero, a rock	Art, Arta, Arte, D'Artagnan
Barry	French, Celtic, Welsh	Spear thrower, son of Harry, Marksman	Barrie, Barris, Barie, Barrymore
Cedric	Welsh	Bounty, spectacle, founder	Cedrick, Cedrych, Cerdric
Clyde	Welsh	Heard from afar	
Conway	Welsh	River, hound of the plain	Conwy
Deverell	Welsh	From the riverbank	
Dewey	Welsh	Devin	
Dewitt	Welsh	Blond	
Dylan	Welsh	Sea god, son of the waves	Dillon, Dillan
Elgan	Welsh	Bright circle	
Emrick	Welsh	Immortal	Emryk, Emrys, Emris
Ffionn	Welsh	Foxglove Flower	
Gareth	Welsh, Norse, Old French	Gentle; enclosure; watchful	Garth, Garret, Garrett, Garreth, Gareth, Garit, Gary, Garry, Gar
Gavin	Welsh	White hawk	Gavan
Gawain	Welsh	Courteous	Gawaine, Gawen
Griffith	Welsh	Fierce chief; ruddy	Griff, Griffie
Iago	Welsh, Spanish	Supplanter	
Kay	Old Welsh, Old German	Rejoicer; fort	Kay, Kai, MacKay
Keith	Celtic; Welsh	Wood, wind; wood-dweller	

Kenn	Welsh	Clear water	
Kenrich	Welsh, Old English	Chief hero; royal ruler	Kenrick, Kenway, Kenley, Kennard
Lloyd	Old Welsh	Gray-haired	Floyd
Maddock	Old Welsh	Champion, good fortune	Madock, Madoc, Madog, Maddox, Madox, Maidoc
Merlin	Celtic, Anglo-Saxon, Welsh	Sea; falcon; sea hill	Merlyn, Marlin, Marlen, Marwin, Mervin, Merv, Merle
Newlyn	Old Welsh	Pool	
Owen	Old Welsh, Greek	Warrior; well born	Owyn, Ewan, Ewen, Owens
Pembroke	Welsh	From the headland, rocky hill	
Perry	Middle English, Welsh	Pear tree; son of Harry	Pierrey, Parry, Perianne, Perian, Perrin, Perin
Powell	Old Welsh	Son of Howell	Powers, Power
Price	Old Welsh	Urgent one	Pryce
Reece	Old Welsh	Enthusiastic	Riece, Reace, Rase, Rice, Rhys, Rhett, Rett
Reese	Welsh	Ardent one	Rhys, Ries
Renfrew	Old Welsh	From the still waters	Renfred, Renshaw, Renton
Sayer	Welsh	Carpenter	Sayers, Sayre, Sayres
Sonnagh	Welsh	Mound, rampart	

Trahaearn	Welsh	Strong as iron	Trahern, Tray
Tristan	Old Welsh, Latin	Noisy one, laborer	Tristram

Yoruban Male Baby Names

Name	Origin	Meaning	Similiar Names
Ajayi	Yoruban, Nigerian	Born face-down	
Bandele	Yoruban	Born away from home	
Kayin	Yoruban	Celebrated child	

- Campbell - 268
- Caleb
- Tegan
- Ian - 274
- Channing
- Willem - 352

Printed in the United States
217025BV00001B/4/A

9 781589 397507